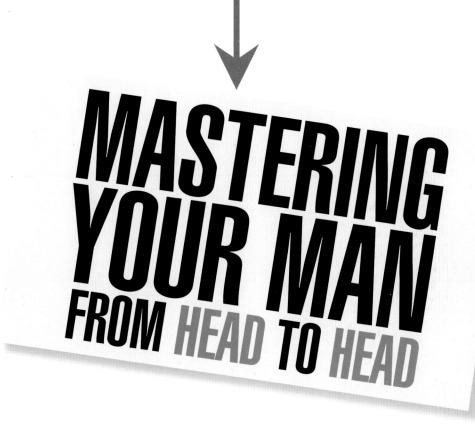

MASTERING YOUR MAN
FROM HEAD TO HEAD

HOW TO WORK YOUR MAN BELOW THE BELT, BETWEEN THE AND BENEATH THE SHEETS FOR **EXCEPTIONAL SEX**

JORDAN LAROUSSE & SAMANTHA SADE

QUIVER

Text © 2010 Yvonne Falvey Mihalik and Naomi Tepper
Photography © 2010 Quiver

First published in the USA in 2010 by
Quiver, a member of
Quayside Publishing Group
100 Cummings Center
Suite 406-L
Beverly, MA 01915-6101
www.quiverbooks.com

14 13 12 11 10   1 2 3 4 5

ISBN-13: 978-1-59233-436-0
ISBN-10: 1-59233-436-9

Library of Congress Cataloging-in-Publication Data
LaRousse, Jordan.
   Mastering your man from head to head : how to work your man below the belt, between the ears, and beneath the sheets for exceptional sex / Jordan LaRousse and Samantha Sade.
      p. cm.
   Includes bibliographical references.
   ISBN-13: 978-1-59233-436-0
   ISBN-10: 1-59233-436-9
   1. Sex instruction for women. 2. Men—Sexual behavior. 3. Sex (Psychology) I. Sade, Samantha. II. Title.
   HQ46.L34 2010
   613.9'6—dc22

                                        2010018223

Cover design by Traffic Design Consultants Ltd.
Book design by Monica Rhines
Illustrations by Robert Brandt

Printed and bound in Singapore

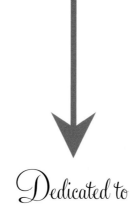

Dedicated to

Brent and Steve. We've enjoyed being your dirty little secret over the years.
Thanks for sharing all of your dirty secrets with us.
And, as always, to Joe.

CONTENTS

GIRL TALK

We were celebrating a best friend's birthday in Breckenridge, Colorado, drinking champagne and eating birthday cake. As usually happens amongst good friends who share a glass of celebratory bubbly, the talk quickly turned to sex. Amid the conspiratorial sharing of techniques and stories, one friend remarked that her boyfriend's cum tastes like Peanut M&Ms, to which another friend responded, "My husband's cum tastes like fresh cucumbers!"

Empowered women everywhere are engaging in conversations like this on their cell phones or over glasses of wine all across the country. We are exploring male sexuality to greater depths, seeking to increase our capacity for pleasure and intimacy. Over brunch with our best friends, we discuss the hottest vibrator on the market (thanks, Oprah!), the new technique we've discovered for giving him amazing oral sex, and how lusty or lackluster our sex lives are at present—and what to do about it!

In writing *Mastering Your Man from Head to Head*, it's our desire to give women just like you a sound education on that sexy creature that we call man, and fill in any gaps in information—those bits of silence, if you will, in the never-ending sex chat between girlfriends. We want to help enable you to take your sex life to the next level. Whether you want to learn a new technique in the bedroom or bring out a whole new sexual side in your partner, this book will give you the tools to do so.

We look forward to pushing the boundaries of sex talk and answering your questions about men (and maybe even a few questions you didn't know you had) including the following: Does every man's cum taste the same? (No!) What on earth should you do with those sexy, sensitive glands he calls nuts? Can an anal-shy guy ever enjoy anal play? Are there any secret spots that will have him melting in your hands? Where does he love to feel your teeth and where does he hate to? Are there any sex toys made for him, and if so, what should you do with them? Filled with techniques, tips, serious information, and even some opinion, this book will help you get to know your man and his every quirk as intimately as you know yourself.

WHY WE USE DIRTY WORDS

Plain and simple: We love them! There's just nothing like the properly timed dirty word, inside the bedroom or out. But moreover, we use words such as *cock*, *pussy*, *balls*, and *fuck* because they correctly and specifically describe what we're writing about with the beauty of real-life terms. We don't say "Please insert your penis into my vagina, honey," and we won't write that way, either.

ALL MEN ARE DIFFERENT—COMMUNICATION IS YOUR #1 ALLY

The truth of this statement hit home during an important conversation about hand jobs. We were polling a large group of women about proper technique, and every single lady had a different tip. It was a bit overwhelming, until we realized that they were all saying the same thing: Ask him! And this is true for more than hand jobs. You can learn all of the techniques and methods you want, but not every man is going to love everything you do the same way. In fact, what might have one guy coming buckets will have another one turning on the TV and telling you he has a headache. If nothing else, we hope that reading this book will teach you to speak up, ask questions, and open the floodgates of sex chat between you and your man. After all, communication is the necessary foundation and backbone not only for an overall fulfilling sex life, but also for your relationships in general.

INFORMATION, FROM HEAD TO HEAD

As much as we know about sex and the male specimen, we couldn't have possibly put together such a thorough guide for women without the invaluable knowledge imparted to us by our panel of experts, the participants in our sex survey, and our candid interviews with real men.

OUR PANEL OF EXPERTS

- **Dr. Emmey Ripoll, M.D.,** is a practicing urologist in Boulder, Colorado. She has published two books and has over thirty publications in the field of urology. Dr. Ripoll is double-certified by the American Board of Urology and the American Board of Integrative Holistic Medicine. A certified yoga instructor and practitioner of Qigong, Dr. Ripoll utilizes acupuncture in the treatment of urological conditions.
- **Dr. Jenni Skyler, Ph.D., MS.Ed.,** is a sex therapist and board-certified sexologist. She is the director of the Intimacy Institute for sex and relationship therapy in Boulder, Colorado. Dr. Skyler also writes the "Sexpress Yourself" column for Datebility.com and is an expert author on SexualHealth.com.
- **Dr. Richard Wagner Ph.D., ACS,** or Dr. Dick, as we fondly know him, is a clinical sexologist based in Seattle, Washington. He's been a practitioner of sex therapy and relationship counseling for more than twenty-five years. For well over a decade, he has been writing the popular "Dr. Dick" sex advice column at www.drdicksexadvice.com.
- **Dr. Glenda Walden, Ph.D.,** has been an instructor in sociology at the University of Colorado, Boulder, since 2003 and currently teaches Social Construction of Sexuality.

THE SEX SURVEY

Using an anonymous sex survey, we gathered intimate information from 491 women and 323 men. The survey was open for several months in 2009. Many participants found the survey link at OystersandChocolate.com, an online magazine for literary erotica, so we must assume that most, if not all, respondents were at least sexually open enough to read erotic short stories. Many of the colorful quotes, statistics, graphs, and charts in the book are extrapolated from this survey, but please keep in mind that we are neither scientists nor professional statisticians.

PERSONAL INTERVIEWS

We had the opportunity to sit down with both men and women and conduct in-depth and blushingly personal interviews about their sex lives and sexual selves. Many quotes and specific examples come from these interviews. But again, this was done informally, and in some cases, large amounts of tequila were involved. Please note that all identifying information for survey respondents and interviewees has been changed, including names, ages, and professions.

COMMON SENSE

Ladies, we've worked our little tails off to provide you with information that is as true and informative and helpful as should be fit to share over the sacred bonds of sisterhood. We don't take this lightly, and we give you the same advice we would offer to our best friends. But please, take into account that we are not medical doctors, we do not have Ph.D.s, nor have we spent countless hours studying and doing experiments in white rooms on poor, helpless men chained to sterile tables with their penises attached to wires and electrodes. In other words, all of this information is subjective, as is life. None of this information should be construed as complete medical advice, nor is it meant to replace the medical advice of your doctor. So use your common sense and decency when dealing with the opposite sex (and when dealing with anyone). If you ever do anything to put yourself at harm or at risk with the law, please know we are not to be held accountable. Ultimately, you are responsible for your sex life. Stay safe and have fun!

LEARN MORE

For further reading on men and sex, we highly recommend the following books:
- *The Guide to Getting It On!* by Paul Joannides
- *Passionista: The Empowered Woman's Guide to Pleasuring a Man*, by Dr. Ian Kerner
- *The New Good Vibrations Guide to Sex*, by Cathy Winks and Anne Semans

$Chapter$ **1**

SAY HELLO TO YOUR LITTLE FRIEND: MR. PENIS

YES, GIRLS, although you might think that a dick is just a dick, when you observe closely, you'll find that the penis is a fascinating piece of equipment. It grows, it shrinks, it changes shape. It is a source of pleasure and a cause of frustration. It is simultaneously both soft and hard, both durable and fragile. It's the anatomical centerpiece of the sexual spread of his body, and as such, it's the first part of his body that we'll address.

As women, we wonder what it would be like to have one of these things dangling between our legs. Of course, we're not talking penis envy, ladies, but something closer to penis curiosity. For example, does a men's size 12 shoe mean he's got a big package? Can you really break his penis? Do uncircumcised men wield a sensation advantage over their cut counterparts? And why do some men name their cocks? We'll investigate these and other questions about that incredible little piece of flesh we call the cock, as well as some of the better ways to reach out and touch one.

SIZE MATTERS (OR MATTERS OF SIZE)

The size of a man's penis has become almost as large a cultural obsession as the size of a woman's breasts. Every day, our spam folders get flooded with emails containing subject lines such as "Women can't find your thing in your pants? Enlarge it." Despite the fact that most women aren't complaining, we can understand how this stuff might get into a guy's head (and for only $199.95 for a six-month supply of herbal enhancers, maybe even into his *head*, too). The good news is that—despite all these questionable emails—pornography featuring big-dicked actors, and other subconscious and pop-culture size messages, 76 percent of our male survey respondents said they are happy with their penis size and 87 percent said they've never tried to change their size. Honestly, we are impressed!

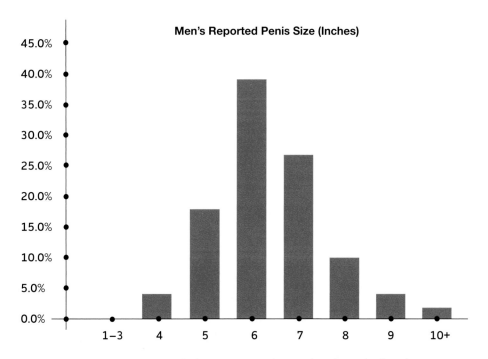

Men's Reported Penis Size (Inches)

In our survey of 285 men, the majority reported having a 6-inch (15.24 cm) penis when erect. Scientists say that the average length of the American man's penis is between 5.25 and 5.5 inches (13.35 and 13.97 cm) when erect.

ARE YOU A GREAT DANE GIRL, OR DO YOU PREFER THE POCKET-PAL CHIHUAHUA?

Remember season two, episode thirty of *Sex and the City* when the hypersexual Samantha meets Mr. Too Big? She decides they are better off friends, for the safety of her vagina. Then later, in season four, episode sixty-one, she meets Richard and reveals, "He's got the most perfect dick I've ever seen. Long, pink, amazing. It's dickalicious!" Much like Samantha, all women have their own idea of penis perfection. But how closely does it relate to size?

In a 2006 *Oysters & Chocolate* reader survey, we asked women to tell us whether size really mattered to them. The results? Yes, size matters—but that doesn't always mean bigger is better. And size isn't the only thing that matters; they also reported preferences on girth, angle, hygiene, circumcision, and more.

Jennifer puts it succinctly, "Of course size matters, but so many things matter more."

THE SCOOP ON HIS HUGE WANG

So what makes a big dick big? Dr. Emmey says that it's basically a matter of hormones. The more growth hormones and androgens your guy had available to him during his adolescence (the most well-known androgen being testosterone), the bigger his penis will be. Men's penises stop growing about the same time their bodies do, typically between the ages of 17 and 21.

Scientists tell us that the average penis size is about 5.5 inches (13.97 cm) when fully erect. That means that a 6- or 7-incher (15.24 or 17.78 cm) is already above average, and a big dick is anything 8 inches (20.32 cm) or longer.

Rumor has it that if your guy has a big dick, he *is* a big dick. Is it true that a man with a swelled head below the belt leads to a man with a swelled head above the neck? Researchers at the School of Psychology at the University of Victoria in Melbourne, Australia, aim to find out. A team led by Dr. Gerard Kennedy has hypothesized that a man with a larger penis will have more confidence and a better body image than his smaller counterpart.[1] As of the writing of this book, the study has not yet been published. But if these researchers have it right, chances are, a guy with a larger-than-life appendage may get a little cocky—that is, if he lets his confidence get the best of him.

Size is a personal preference, and some women truly love big dicks. Laura, 37, says it well: "In terms of pleasure and sex appeal, size does matter. . . . There are some people who simply are turned on by seeing a large penis . . . seeing someone who is well-endowed is similar to hearing someone who sings exceptionally well or dances well. . . . It is not the norm, and so you are attracted to that which is unique."

But it's not always romance and excitement with a well-endowed man. If you were ever (un)lucky enough to see the Tommy Lee and Pamela Anderson sex tape, you witnessed what happens when two bodies don't quite fit together. Pamela couldn't take Tommy's whole package, and what looks painful for her looks unsatisfying for him.

The ouch factor created when a man bumps his super-sized penis up against your cervix during intercourse is no fun (the doggy-style position is the worst culprit). Anal sex is often out of the question with well-endowed guys. And oral sex can be difficult; you may have trouble wrapping your mouth around his girth, and if he does manage to get in deep you may have an issue with your gag reflex.

Dr. Jenni says:

"To properly measure his erect penis, start at the base where the testicles connect to the shaft and measure the length of the underside. For a man who usually measures at the topside of his shaft, he may be surprised that he's miraculously gained an inch!"

For some women, these setbacks are considered challenges that they'll happily surmount (or mount!). So for those of you who may have one of these trophy dicks to hang on your wall, we have one word for you: lubrication. Check out chapter 7, "Toys for Boys," for more info on what type of lube to use.

TIDBITS ON THE TEENY WEENIE

Okay, so let's say you unwrap a guy's banana and find that the fruit is about the size of an appetizer at a fancy French restaurant. What's a girl to do? Although size doesn't matter when a guy is within the average zone, let's be honest here: An extra-small package can matter a lot to some women.

Our culture has a very narrow-minded view of sex, often defining it exclusively as the act of penetration of penis into vagina. President Bill Clinton argued for this classic definition of sex when he firmly pronounced "I did not have sexual relations with that woman!" He said this despite the fact that Monica Lewinsky had given him blow jobs, and he in turn had penetrated his intern with a cigar. Does this mean that oral sex isn't sex when it's a blow job and penetration isn't sex when it's done using an object instead of a boner? We think we should redefine *sex* to mean "the mutual sensual exploration of your partner's body (or partners' bodies!)." That would solve a lot of problems (and "Slick Willies" wouldn't get away with playing word games).

So what does this have to do with a teeny weenie? If penetration alone will not satisfy, finding yourself entangled in the bed sheets with a hotty sporting a wee woody does not have to be a disappointing experience. Now is your opportunity to explore that "other kind of sex" where penetration is but a cherry on the cupcake.

Tips for Loving a Petite Penis

- Break out the sex toys and explore each other in new ways.
- Spend more time enjoying oral sex (his and hers).
- Test the boundaries of anal sex.
- Make love to his entire body and allow him to do the same to yours.
- Encourage your guy to do his kegels. This won't enlarge his penis, but it will strengthen it, which could improve his stamina and confidence.
- Try a cock ring. This toy will temporarily increase his penis size.

You may find that in letting go of your penis-centricity, you'll experience sex in novel ways that you may have never before imagined. Also remember that your vagina is most sensitive to touch on the labia, the clitoris, and the first three inches of the interior canal. The rest of the tunnel is sensitive to pressure, which explains why you may enjoy deep penetration but not need it to orgasm.

Says Joy, "Yes, size matters to me. Brain size. . . . But cock size? Never. I seldom have penetrative orgasms. Mine are clitoral and cerebral."

THE AVERAGE JOE

The truth is, most guys reside in the neither-too-big-nor-too-small category. In our survey, 18 percent of men reported a 5-inch (12.7 cm) erection and 39 percent reported having a 6-incher (15.24 cm). Chances are, the men you meet will have members of a moderate proportion.

Straddling an average Joe will usually make for perfectly pleasurable sex. We recommend lavishing your guy (big, small, or in between) with plenty of ego-boosting compliments about his johnson. It's great for his body image and self-esteem, just as great as when your guy compliments your bubble butt, gorgeous face, and pretty toes.

Sandra says, "So, does size matter? Yes, it does. Middle-sized, that's the thing—not too big and not too small. As long as he knows what he's doing, then Mr. Average is, for me, Mr. Perfect."

SIZE MYTH #1: DO BIG HANDS MEAN BIG DICKS?

As women, we've all heard the comment "Oooh, big hands (or feet)—you know what that means, wink wink." For some reason, we women are obsessed with trying to guess the size of a guy's dick before we even pull his pants down. Because it's unlikely that we'll be able to undress every man we meet who has big feet, we wanted to get to the bottom of this myth.

After evaluating 285 male respondents who answered questions regarding the size of their hands, feet, and erect cocks, we found absolutely no correlation between the size of the penis and that of the other appendages. The majority of men reported having a 6-inch (15.24 cm), fully erect penis, and most men also reported wearing size 10 sneakers. However, these two numbers did not directly relate. A man with a 4-inch (10.16 cm) cock was shown to be as likely as the man with the 9-incher (22.86 cm) to wear a size 10 shoe. Additionally, men with all sizes of penises reported that they had been told they have big hands.

Our unscientific study is backed up by a scientific one undertaken in 2002 by the Department of Urology at St. Mary's Hospital and the Institute of Urology at University College Hospitals in London. A team of curious doctors enlisted the help of 104 men who agreed to come into a clinic where researchers would compare their shoe sizes with their penis sizes. The scientists benefited from having a hands-on test, instead of one where the men simply reported their sizes. However, the M.D.s didn't want to get their gloves dirty handling erections. So they simply made sure the room was warm enough to prevent shrinkage and then stretched the poor subjects' flaccid penises out to full length and measured them. The results: "The median stretched penile length for the sampled population was 5.11 inches (12.97 cm) and the median U.S. shoe size was 10. There was no statistically significant correlation between shoe size and stretched penile length."[2]

This myth is busted!

SIZE MYTH #2: DOES SIZE VARY BY CULTURE?

The stereotype of the black man's larger-than-average endowment goes back centuries. A German anthropologist named Johann Friedrich Blumenbach said in 1795, "It is generally said that the penis of the Negro is very large. And this assertion is so far borne out by the remarkable genital apparatus of an Ethiopian which I have in my anatomical collection."[3] Yes you read that correctly, this guy collected penises! How he got them, we really don't want to know.

More recently, a number of studies have been conducted to try to determine who wins the "biggest penis" prize, but they all seem to contradict each other greatly in their results. Dr. Emmey tells us that racial difference in size is, on average, statistically provable, but only when men are flaccid. Any visible differences are nullified when men develop erections.

The folks at the Kinsey Institute explain how this could be so: "There is a much wider range of size in men's penises when flaccid, with the average ranging from 1 to 4 inches (2.54 to 10.16 cm). In general, smaller flaccid penises lengthen at erection by a greater percentage than do larger flaccid penises, with most men reaching an average size of 5 to 7 inches (12.7 to 17.78 cm), so the flaccid size of a penis is not a good predictor of erect size."[4] In short, once those peckers are filled with blood, it's anyone's game.

In any case, does it really matter—especially in this day and age in the United States where race is becoming an ever fuzzier classification? The U.S. Census Bureau's 2006–2008 American Community Survey reported 6.5 million people of multiracial heritage living in the United States (2 percent of the overall population).[5] The lesson? It's probably best not to try to guess your date's penis size by the color of his skin.

This myth is busted!

PENIS SHAPES

Although the slight majority of our survey respondents report having penises that are straight as arrows, 48 percent described their dicks as dangling at different angles.

Describe the "Angle of Your Dangle"

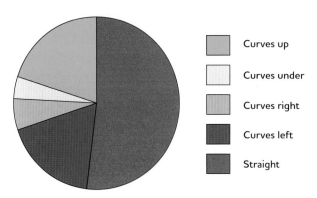

- Curves up
- Curves under
- Curves right
- Curves left
- Straight

As with intricate snowflakes, no two cocks are the same. Straight, curved, crooked, or hooked, bulbous, sinuous, thick, or slender—there are about as many shapes of cocks as there are men. For all you ladies who are into sampling and haven't settled on a single mister for the moment, we challenge you to really examine the variety of penises you'll find attached to your variety of lovers. Or view them from a safe distance by watching a porn film, or two, or three.

The thing about cocks is that, just like breasts, nearly every shape (and size) under the sun is normal and healthy.

When erect, your guy's penis will change not only in size, but also shape and sometimes even angle. Says 40-something Jeff, "My penis curves right when soft and it curves up when hard."

Sometimes a man's particular angle can be a perfect match for your own particularly shaped interior space. Says Angela, 37, "What really matters to me is where his penis makes contact. In other words, I need a man who bends to the left. That's the guy who rubs me the right way!"

PENILE PHENOMENA

They do seem to have a mind of their own, don't they? In this section we'll discuss a variety of common penile behaviors that can be baffling to those of us without sausage-shaped genitalia.

MORNING WOOD

We're sure you've experienced it: You roll over in bed to snuggle with your guy in the morning only to find that he already has an erection. This erection is not there because he's dreaming about sex, so you should probably ask his opinion about early morning sex before you hop on top. In our survey, 90 percent of the men we asked said they love morning sex—but make sure your guy doesn't fall into the minority who does not. Tim, a 22-year-old student, says he likes it "because she just looks so damn hot in the morning. I also like having sex when we take our morning shower together."

Rob, a 30-something attorney, says he likes it "because my wife hasn't had anything to be mad at me about yet."

But 50-something Ray tells us he's not into morning lovin' because "I'm old and I have to pee when I wake up."

Dr. Emmey says:

"The first thing I ask a man who comes in complaining about erectile dysfunction (ED) is, 'Do you have morning erections?' If he does, his ED is more likely a result of an emotional problem. If he doesn't, it's a definite sign of a physiological problem. It could be a problem with hormones, arterial or venous supply, diabetes . . . a whole host of possible health issues."

A healthy man will experience erections approximately three to five times per night, during the REM cycles of his sleep, and he should experience morning erections for his entire life.

PREMATURE EJACULATION (TAKE COVER!)

Loosely defined, premature ejaculation (PE) is simply ejaculating during sex sooner than a man and his partner (you) would like. This can become a problem if it occurs with some consistency. The Mayo Clinic estimates that as many as one in three men may be affected by PE at some time in his life.[6]

PE is a hard issue to pin down because "premature" varies for each person and each couple. For some couples, being able to have intercourse for two to three minutes before he ejaculates would be just dandy. For others, ejaculating before a minimum of thirty minutes might be unacceptable (lucky ducks!).

The causes of PE range from being wholly medical to being completely psychological. For the more serious cases of PE, such as the man who comes at a simple brush of the hand or the guy who comes after only one or two strokes inside his lover (they don't call him the three-pump chump for nothing!), there are a wide range of treatment options. The professional consensus seems to be that a combination of undergoing psychological/sexual counseling, practicing sexual techniques while solo and with a partner, and even taking medications will deliver the best results for serious PE.

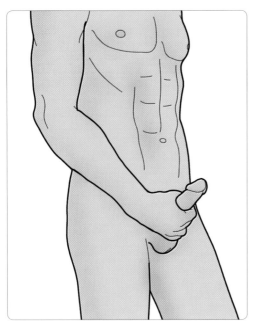

If your lover simply wants to last longer and doesn't need professional help, there are some fun exercises that can be done solo or together. "One of the biggest sexual complaints for younger male patients is that they come too fast (Premature Ejaculation). PE is such an easy fix. The start-stop technique is one of the basic techniques taught," says Dr. Jenni.

Your man can practice the start-stop method solo as he learns to overcome premature ejaculation.

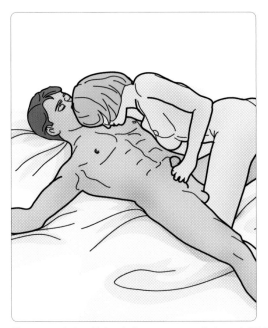
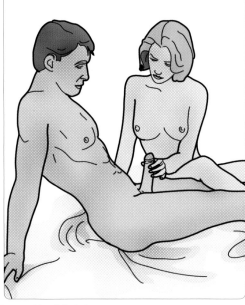

Use a a gentle hand job to help your man work through PE. Squeeze him right below the cockhead when you want him to slow down.

Tips and Techniques for Making Him Last

- First, Dr. Jenni recommends that a man identify a scale of arousal from 1 to 10, where 1 is flaccid and 10 is ejaculation. This means that 9 would be the point where ejaculation is inevitable, which would make 8 the key "stop" point, and 3 or 4 the "start again" points.
- Encourage your lover to masturbate during the week and practice taking himself up to an 8 and back down again to a 3 or 4 at least three times before he brings himself to ejaculation. (Men trying this for the first time may want to do this solo and try out going only up to a 6 or 7 at first.)
- Give your lover a nice, slow hand job. Ask him to tell you when he has reached an 8 (you may be able to tell this yourself if you know him well enough). Then squeeze your thumb and forefinger just below the ridge of his cock head (at the corona). Do this for about 30 seconds, then proceed with your hand job. Do this a few times before you let him ejaculate.

- Try practicing this technique of taking him to an 8 and back down with what Dr. Jenni calls "the quiet vagina," which means that when he comes to a stopping point during sex, you don't move your body or your vaginal muscles at all. Once this is mastered you can try having him stop within "the active vagina."

Obviously, girls, the most important thing with these techniques is practice, practice, practice. What fun! The more your lover gets to know his own levels of arousal and control moving through them, up, down, and back again, the longer he'll be able to go before ejaculating.

PENISES ARE SPRAINABLE AND BREAKABLE

If there aren't any real bones in a boner, how can it be broken? Dr. Emmey tells us that men can experience acute penile fractures, often as a result of slipping out during intercourse and accidentally ramming his rod into your pubic bone. This unhappy accident very often occurs when a woman is on top. Ouch! If this happens and you hear a popping sound, you may have broken a ligament in his penis. Most likely, his penis will bend in an odd direction and become black and blue. It's important to get him to the ER for immediate attention if this happens.

Dr. Emmey tells us that a man can also experience chronic micro fractures throughout his lifetime (possibly as a result of having sex when he isn't fully erect, accidentally bending his penis as he inserts it). Calcification builds up around the fractures, and Dr. Emmey says that if he accumulates enough of these calcifications, it can lead to Peyronie's disease down the road. Peyronie's is a painful and severe bend (often 90 degrees or worse) in the penis that prevents a man from leading a healthy sex life.

THE PENIS NAME GAME

The old joke goes, "Do you know why a man gives his penis a nickname? To prevent a complete stranger from making all of his decisions for him." It turns out that 18 percent of the men we surveyed named their penises, while 38 percent of women surveyed reported that they've been with a partner whose penis has a name. The most common names? Mister Happy, Junior, Richard, Woody, and Little *insert his name here*. The strangest account came from Lucy, who said, "It happened to be my mother's name!"

AMUSING PENIS NAMES

- Bruce (as in Bruce Lee)
- Der Fuhrer (because he's a blitzkrieg of penile perfection and prowess)
- Narsil (from *Lord of the Rings*)
- Lil' Elvis
- Energizer (he keeps going and going)
- Big Ben
- The Hammer of Israel
- The Duck
- Maxwell (from the Maxwell House commercial: good to the last drop)
- His Majesty
- George (one man named it after the father of our country)
- Wilber the One-Eyed Wonder Worm

- Arnold (named after the California governor)
- Bone Daddy the Magnificent
- Princess Sophie (your guess is as good as ours on this one)
- Weapon of Mass Satisfaction
- Mr. Hamster
- The White Stallion (versus the Black Stallion)
- Troy the Love Toy
- General (this one changed when it got promoted)
- The Moccasin
- Wally (and the Beaver . . .)
- Trouble
- Shorty Chorizo
- Willie Wonka
- Super Freak

Some men have perfectly logical reasons for naming this appendage. Says 30-something Zach, "It allows us to talk about sex in front of the kids without letting on." Others were romantically dubbed in times of war. Says Harry, a 50-something U.S. Army General, "At one time I was stationed overseas and my wife was in the States. When I would send her a letter, I signed it from me and 'Richard.' It let her know that I missed her sexually, in addition to emotionally. I had to have something to call it besides from me and my cock!"

Yet others shared humorous stories. Says 40-something Lenny, "As a freshman in college, the other guys were talking about these guys I'd never met. After a few such moments, I realized they were talking about their penises, and called them out on it. 'You named your dicks?' Yes, they said. 'That's ridiculous. And if you're going to name them, why not name them something worthy, like, I dunno, Wotan, Father of Gods?' They broke up over that, but thenceforth I was the proud bearer of Wotan."

For many men, the women they are with are the naming culprits; indeed, 11 percent of the women we surveyed told us they helped pick the name. Says 50-something Ron, "My ex—who was absolutely great in bed—named it J.R. after the character in the *Dallas* TV show. I never called it anything but ready."

But not all men have boarded the name train. In fact, a great number of the men we polled were insulted at the very thought of giving a body part a name. Says 44-year-old Luke, "It's a part of me. Contrary to popular belief, it does *not* have a mind of its own."

CIRCUMCISION UNCUT ▶

Usually the "to snip or not to snip" question is answered by your man's parents long before he becomes your lover. Every baby boy is born with a foreskin; circumcision is the quick operation in which the foreskin is removed. In the United States, approximately 60 percent to 70 percent of men are circumcised, as compared to 15 percent of men worldwide. And indeed, in our survey 76 percent of our respondents said they are circumcised; many of those who replied that they're uncut are from the United Kingdom, where circumcision is no longer a common practice.

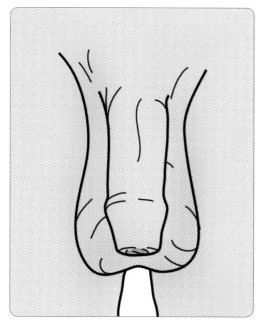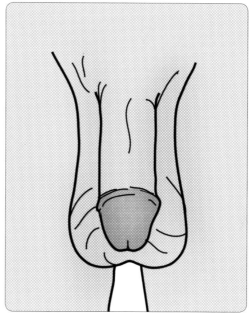

When flaccid, the head of the uncircumcised penis (left) is covered by the foreskin, while the head of the circumcised penis (right) is exposed.

THE CIRCUMCISION PROCEDURE

In the United States, circumcisions are usually performed during the first month of life, if not within the first few days. If done in the hospital, the doctor cleans the baby's penis and foreskin, a special clamp is attached to the penis, and the foreskin is quickly snipped away. Ointment and gauze or some other type of sterile protection is then put on the little guy to keep it from rubbing against the diaper. The procedure is quick, and some doctors even provide a local anesthetic.

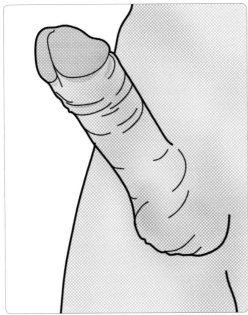
When erect, the head of the uncircumcised penis becomes exposed as the foreskin retracts.

REASONS FOR CIRCUMCISION

Circumcision has been a practice all over the world for thousands of years. According to Robert Darby, B.A., B.Litt., Ph.D., circumcision was practiced as a puberty rite among the Aborigines as long ago as 10,000 BCE. Tribes in northeastern Africa and on the Arabian peninsula did likewise around 6,000 BCE. In 600 BCE, the reference to Yahweh's command to Abraham to circumcise himself as well as his sons and the rest of the males in the household was immortalized in the book of Genesis. Around 450 BCE, Greek historians noted that circumcision, as well as other penile mutilations, were prevalent among Arabs and other Middle Eastern tribes.[7]

Different peoples took up and abandoned the practice of circumcision for several hundred years. However, the present-day attitudes in the United States regarding circumcision have roots dating back to the medical field of the nineteenth century. Influential doctors, such as French physician Claude François Lallemand, James Copland, and John Harvey Kellogg (yes, of the cereal fame), promoted circumcision as a deterrent for masturbation. These antimasturbation ideas were embraced in Britain, Australia, and the United States, but not in Europe.

Other arguments for circumcision have included the rate of transmission of sexually transmitted infections (STIs)—from the 1800s, when physicians argued that circumcised boys were less likely to contract syphilis, to the more recent, controversial studies suggesting that male circumcision reduces the risk of men's HIV infection during sex with women. Still other organizations and studies have suggested that uncircumcised men have higher rates of penile cancer, and their partners have higher rates of cervical cancer. However, all of these claims and studies have been refuted as inconclusive or methodically flawed.

THE JOYS OF AN UNCIRCUMCISED COCK

For a variety of reasons, it appears that the foreskin has been demonized in Western countries (specifically the United States, Britain, and Australia) over the past couple hundred years. Whether it was responsible for the evils of masturbation, disseminating syphilis, causing cancer, or spreading HIV, one medical expert or another has attempted to again take up the call for the mass practice of circumcision.

The reality? Most research suggests that the foreskin is simply a part of the penis that has gotten a bad rap. Indeed, the American Academy of Pediatrics has stated and restated since 1975 that "there is no absolute medical indication for routine circumcision of the newborn."

G-Spot Stimulation ▼

You would be hard-pressed to see a difference between a circumcised penis and an uncircumcised one when each is erect. How can this be so? With arousal, the foreskin pulls back to bear the cock's head uncovered, rendering it visually similar to its snipped counterpart. However, many women insist that when an uncircumcised man is hard, his foreskin creates a larger ridge, or corona, which rubs oh-so-nicely against the G-spot during intercourse. Thus, it is often lovingly referred to as the G-spot stimulator.

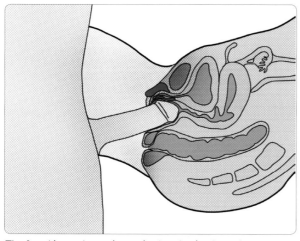

The foreskin on the uncircumcised cock stimulates the g-spot.

"I've been with both circumcised and uncircumcised men, and I've noticed a difference with G-spot stimulation," says Jane, a 30-something literary agent. "With an uncut lover, the foreskin forms a type of ridge right behind the head of the penis, and I can feel it on my G-spot when he strokes in and out of me. It makes it much easier for him to get the right spot, and I am much more likely to have an orgasm during sex when the man is uncircumcised."

Natural Lubrication

When we think of circumcision, the issue of lubrication doesn't often come to mind. However, it turns out that natural lubrication is a whole different animal when it comes to sex with an intact man. The foreskin has a self-cleansing, mucosal membrane, similar to the membranes on the inner eyelids and the vagina, which provides natural lubrication that allows the foreskin to easily move up and down the shaft during both masturbation and intercourse.[8] The foreskin also serves to capture more of the woman's natural lubrication and keep it present during intercourse. The result? A lot more lubrication inside the vagina during sex. Says Ali, 38, "I've noticed much less chaffing and irritation with my uncircumcised lovers, even when having sex multiple times in a row or in one day. It's also easier to have sex in wet conditions, such as in the shower, Jacuzzi, or pool, as my natural wetness is less likely to be washed away." Suze, a 42-year-old project manager, puts it more simply: "Sex is silkier and wetter with uncircumcised men."

Cock Sensitivity

It is becoming a widely held belief that an intact man's cock is actually more sensitive than a circumcised man's.

Says 50-something Ruth, "The majority of my lovers have been uncircumcised, and there are definitely differences between cut and uncut penises. Whereas many men with circumcised penises require hard, fast movements (like 'beating off' or 'pounding' their partner) to get off, the uncircumcised penis is way more sensitive and is more easily stimulated by small movements and light touch. When I give an uncircumcised man head, I can drive him wild by running my tongue and fingers over his head and retracted foreskin, lightly licking and caressing him. Fellatio is a more delicate process overall, and I don't feel like a Hoover with endless sucking and whacking to get him off."

There appears to be conflicting scientific information on the sensitivity issue. A study published in *BJU International* in April 2007 found that five locations on the uncircumcised penis that are routinely removed at circumcision are more sensitive than the most sensitive part of the circumcised penis. The overall conclusion was that "the glans of the circumcised penis is less sensitive to fine touch than the glans of the uncircumcised penis. Circumcision ablates (removes) the most sensitive parts of the penis."[9]

However, a different study undertaken by Kimberley Pane Ph.D. et al., of the Riverside Professional Center in Ottawa, Canada, says the opposite. These researchers argued that other studies failed to bring their subjects to arousal before testing for sensitivity. To rectify this oversight, this study had forty men—twenty of whom were uncircumcised—watch an erotic film. They then measured penile sensitivity to touch and pain. Their results stated that "No differences in genital sensitivity were found between the uncircumcised and circumcised groups." Although, oddly, they also reported that "Uncircumcised men were less sensitive to touch on the forearm than circumcised men."[10] What arms have to do with penises, we do not know.

In all practicality, determining which man's penis feels sex more acutely is a tall order. It's such a subjective experience, and one that would be infinitely difficult to compare—even if you ask "Hey, honey, does your penis feel more excited than my ex-boyfriend's did?" We do know one thing, however: Healthy men, both cut and uncut, love sex. Period.

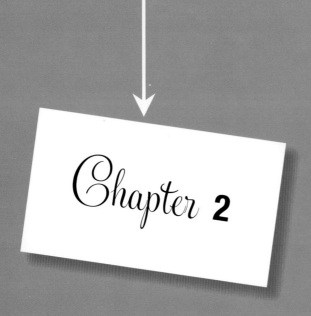

Chapter **2**

THE TESTICLES: DELIVERING PLEASURE DOWN UNDER

ON THE OUTSIDE, testicles may seem like secondary playthings to be touched or licked in passing on your way to pleasuring the big kahuna; but on the inside, these guys could arguably occupy the center ring in the three-ring circus. Of course, every little hormonal gland is inextricably important when it comes to the male reproductive system, but the testicles are the primary male reproductive glands.

The scrotum, the contact point at which you will experience your lover's testicles, is the sac that hangs from the penis and embraces the gonads. The outer layer of the scrotum consists of a thin layer of wrinkled skin that covers another layer containing muscle. A thin, internal membrane separates the two testes, keeping them nice and snug in their own little condominiums. The scrotum has its own thermostat, and according to how cold or hot your man may get, the scrotal muscles will pull the testes up or let them hang free.[11]

The testes are responsible for sperm production as well as hormone production. Each testicle contains around 1,000 tiny, compressed tubes, called seminiferous tubules. Amazingly, each tube is 1–3 feet (0.3–0.9 m) long, and if all of the tubes in a man's testicles were laid end to end, they would stretch out to several hundred yards.[12] It is in these many folds of tubes that the production of sperm takes place. It takes about seventy-two days for each little sperm to mature. A man can produce up to 12 trillion sperm during his lifetime, and approximately 400 million are launched from the safety of the penis each time a man ejaculates.

Spermatozoa are all well and good, especially if you're looking to conceive a child. However, the oh-so-much-more-necessary element, a key to the basic upkeep of the machine that is man, is the production of testosterone. And yes, ladies, the testes are where the majority of this happens. The Leydig cells, found within the connective tissues in the testicles, are the tiny manufacturing plants that produce testosterone, as well as other male hormones.[13]

Technically speaking, each testicle is olive-shaped and weighs about 1 ounce (28 g). The testicles are almost never symmetrical, and usually one hangs lower than the other (in 75 percent of men, the left testes hangs lower than the right).[14]

THE IMPORTANCE OF TESTOSTERONE

In pop culture, testosterone gets a bad rap. When you think of testosterone, you think of muscle-bound, iron-pumping idiots. Or you picture hypersexual "playahs" just trying to get you into bed. Most people associate testosterone with the male sex drive or overly masculine features. However, as Dr. Emmey stresses, "Testosterone is incredibly important for men. It's not just about sexual function; it's about insulin resistance, cholesterol, and more."

Let's take a step back and consider the facts. Here are some of the important functions that the superhero testosterone plays a part in and regulates:

- Creation of a lower, manly voice
- Body hair growth (including that beard or goatee you love so much)
- Bone growth
- Increase of muscle mass

- Regulation of cholesterol
- Enhancement of the immune system
- Oxygen uptake

There is also evidence that testosterone helps in mental concentration, improving mood, and preventing depression and perhaps Alzheimer's disease. In addition, it speeds up certain metabolic processes, such as cell production and cell growth.

STRANGE TESTICULAR BEHAVIOR

For the half of the species that doesn't have them, testicles can seem like strange characters indeed. They pull up, they tighten, they shrink, and they're so very sensitive. What's behind all of the simultaneous action and vulnerability?

Think of the testes as the male version of the ovaries, to a certain extent. The testes produce sperm; the ovaries produce ovum (eggs). Also, both are endocrine glands, producing hormones that are directly secreted into the blood. Imagine the logistics of having your ovaries hanging outside of the body!

The testicles are in fact outside of the body to keep the spermatozoa at a nice three to five degrees cooler than body temp (98.6°F [37°C]), because they simply can't survive for very long at body temperature. However, they can't get too cold either, which accounts for "shrinkage"—the phenomenon that occurs when a man has suddenly leaped into a pool of cold water: His testicles pull up into the body to keep the sperm warm. Men experience shrinkage when they're scared as well—again, simply a biological defense mechanism.

As you may have noticed, a man's lovely gonads also pull up during arousal, which helps protect them during the vigorous activity that is sex.[15] And during ejaculation, they tighten and pull up even more, which according to Dr. Emmey, is simply part of the entire pelvic musculature tightening up.

And if you've ever wondered why it hurts men so much when the family jewels take a hit: "Imagine someone striking you in the ovaries! The testicles are like ovaries, but the poor guys are outside the body," says Dr. Emmey. Ouch indeed!

BLUE BALLS . . . FACT OR MYTH?

We've all heard of them, and chances are, you've been with a man or two who has used the term as a negotiation piece in trying to get you to go "all the way." Blue balls, as some men have claimed, is a very painful sensation in the testicles, sometimes accompanied by a bluish color, that is the result of being aroused without then experiencing the climactic joy of ejaculation. So what's the scoop? Is "blue balls" a real thing, or a well-played (and rehearsed) myth?

If a man experiences intense sexual arousal without ejaculation, he may feel a heaviness or some discomfort in the testicles. However, the sensation is far from actual pain, and the feeling will disperse after rest.[16] Dr. Dick tells us that this condition is known as vasocongestion, or the congestion of blood vessels. It's actually a normal part of sexual arousal—for example, it's behind those things we enjoy like erect penises and hard nipples.

Women, too, can be the objects of this affliction, sometimes, but rarely, citing a pain in the pelvis that feels like mild menstrual cramps. The vernacular term for this is *blue walls*. So next time you are feeling dissatisfied, feel free to whine, "But Bob, you *have* to go down on me, or I'll get blue walls!"

Fortunately, the testicular discomfort is very easy to relieve. The first remedy is ejaculation (hence, the pleading cry for help). Other methods include the proverbial cold shower, or just resting and allowing the arousal to recede.

Through practices such as Tantra, men are able to separate orgasm from ejaculation, so that they actually experience small orgasms without ejaculation. To avoid pain in the testicles from a prolonged delay in ejaculation, Tantric lovers sometimes engage in testicular massage during sex, which is said to keep the blood flowing and discomfort at bay.

That said, Dr. Emmey reports that she has never encountered a case of blue balls in her professional career—and in fact, she didn't even know what the term *blue balls* referred to until we explained it. That's a clear indication that the condition is not serious and won't have him running to the ER or even the urologist's office. So if you're not in the mood, just tell your guy to hit the showers (he can decide for himself whether to run the water cold or to use the privacy to ejaculate unaided).

Ladies, the blue balls fact is confirmed, but with a caveat! Blue balls as a seriously painful condition is incredibly rare. The pressure that is more typically felt doesn't warrant serious concern for his health or well-being, so don't ever allow him to use it as a manipulation tool!

TESTACULAR FUN

Testicles are vehicles for all kinds of spectacular erotic pleasure and play (we suppose this is one negative aspect to having the ovaries *inside* the abdomen). Tickling and cupping, licking and sucking are just some of the things you can do to the testicles to have your man moaning for more.

TICKLING AND CUPPING ▼

If you're in the mood to take the reins and seduce your man, the testicles can be key players in his pleasure. Have him lie down on his back, in the nude. Get comfortable sitting between his legs, and lightly brush your fingertips up and down his thighs. Slowly move inward, caressing his inner thighs. Veer around the crotch area, up over his abdomen, and back down again. Let your fingers go higher if you like, over the nipples, along his chest, and over his collarbone. But keep your touch light. When you do decide to brush back down and make contact with his special man parts, concentrate first on the testicles. Outline his testes with your fingers. Tickle them. Cup them and lift

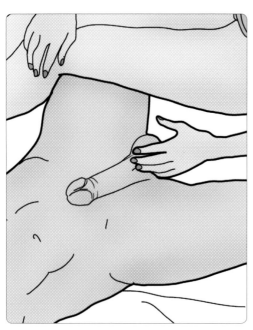
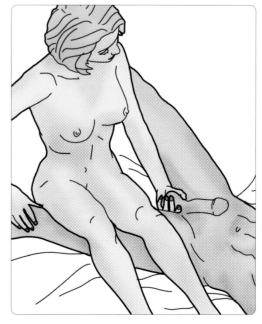

Sit between his legs and tickle and cup his balls.

them, gently. Lean down and exhale slowly, allowing the warm breath from your lips to caress them. Paying such gentle, tantalizing attention to his testes will provide just the right amount of tease and pleasure—and it will set the stage for some intense, intimate time together.

LICKING AND SUCKING ▼

As a sensuous setup for an amazing blow job, lick your way up his inner thighs to his testicles. Some men like long, wet licks along their balls, while others love how it feels to have one testicle gently sucked into the warm, wet confines of your mouth, followed by the other. And some just love it when (and if) you can pull both into your mouth. Do this with loose lips and broad tongue: You never want to force his dynamic duo into a painful squeeze. It's important here to ask what he likes, because one false move with these sensitive little guys can truly put a halt to any sexy plans you may have. Licking and sucking his testicles are excellent ways to slow the blow job down and make it more sensuous. And your mouth on his balls is an amazing way to spice up a hand job.

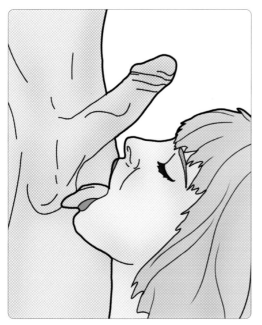
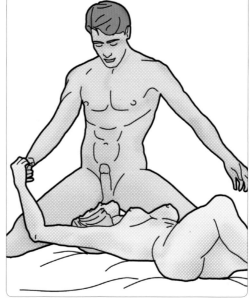

Lick and gently suck his balls into your mouth.

MASSAGE ▼

A slow, soft rub is an incredible turn-on for some men. Roll his testicles with the palm of your hand with broad, circular, gentle motions. You can also incorporate his cock into the massage by brushing the whole of your hand from the bottom of his scrotum and up until you reach the tip of his cock. Draw your hand down along the same path, and repeat.

STRETCHING ▼

Some men love the feel of having their scrotum "stretched." Note here that you're not actually pulling his testicles, but pulling the skin that contains them. Take a solid grip, without pinching, and gently but firmly pull in a downward direction. This movement done intermittently during ball massage, or even a hand job or blow job, will convey the notion that not only are you in charge, but you also know what you're doing. He'll be putty in your hands. Dr. Dick recommends stretching the scrotum especially after a hot shower or bath, which will make the skin more pliable.

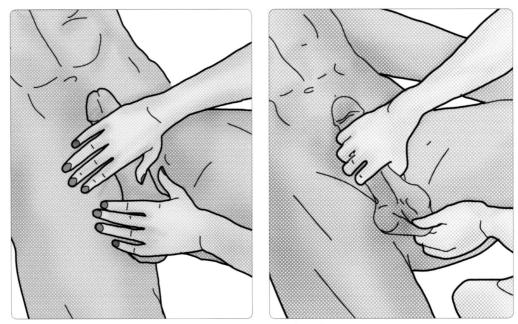

Start with a testicle massage and then gently pull and stretch the skin of his scrotum.

$\mathcal{D}r. \mathcal{D}ick$ *says:*

"The only thing that screams male virility and potency as much as a big dick is a pair of big low-hangin' nuts. In fact, in many societies throughout history a man's cajones were considered sacred. They were revered as objects of religious, social, cultural, and even magical power. In ancient Rome, when a man would take an oath, he would grab his balls, just like we put our hand on a bible today. That's where we got the word *testify*, from the Latin *testis*."

 A TIP ON THE TESTES

Most women think that the base of the penis sits right above where the scrotum hangs, but this isn't true. The base of the cock goes down behind the testicles. To reach and massage this part of his cock, press one of your fingers, length-wise, up into the middle of his scrotum. Use soft, slow pressure and separate his testicles until you get to the base of the scrotum. By pressing here, you are actually pressing an often-untouched part of his penis. If he enjoys it, gently rub back and forth.

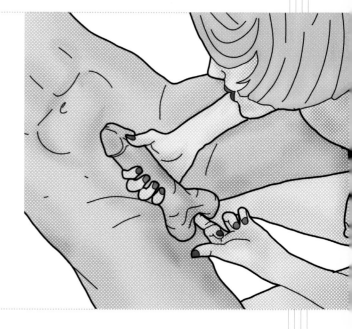

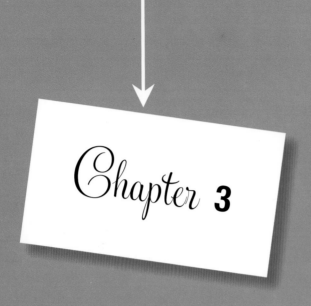

Chapter 3

HOW TO GIVE A BREATHTAKING BLOW JOB

ALSO KNOWN AS FELLATIO, a hummer, a BJ, smoking pole, slob of the knob, giving head, and sucking dick, the blow job is a staple ingredient in a healthy sexual diet. The term is used to describe the sex act of using one's mouth to suck on a man's penis. So why isn't it called a suck job? Your guess is as good as ours!

M. D. Sutton wrote, "One explanation ties the phrase to the jazz slang blow meaning 'to play an instrument.' From there you get the semantic connection of working a tool with some skill, presumably involving the mouth, and there you go. . . . The second school of thought proposes that the blow in blow job indicates the climax and is also related to the expression 'to blow off steam.' Although the phrase blow job dates only from the 1940s, there is a reference to blowing (someone) off, roughly equivalent to the modern phrase getting (someone) off, in David W. Maurer's 1939 glossary, Prostitutes and Criminal Argots."[17]

Once reserved for the bedrooms of prostitutes and gay men, the blow job finally made its way into popular straight culture in the latter part of the twentieth century. In his 2006 *Vanity Fair* article "American as Apple Pie," Christopher Hitchens writes, ". . . the big breakthrough occurs in the great year of nineteen *soixante-neuf*, when Mario Puzo publishes *The Godfather* and Philip Roth brings out *Portnoy's Complaint*. . . . Earthquake! Sensation! Telephones trilled all over the English-speaking world. . . . What is that? And why on earth is it called a 'blow job'? . . . Most of all, notice that it is regular sex that has become obvious and childish, while oral sex is suddenly for real men." [18]

Since the blow job "breakthrough," the term has continued to shed its taboo cloak and openly make its way into the beds of straight couples, the Oval Office, the conversations of many a girls' night out, and men's locker room banter. It's become a technique that any sexually confident woman should know and love.

What makes the blow job so special? Giving one is an act of selfless pleasure, it adds variety to your sex life, and it is a turn-on for all involved!

Dr. Dick says:

"Let's start with the basics. There's no one best way to make oral love to a boner. No two cocksuckers do it exactly the same way, but all have one thing in common, and that's the desire to satisfy. Technique and position take a back seat to simply craving a cock in your mouth. We're not talkin' rocket science, girlfriend; it's just a pecker and a mouth doin' what comes natural. So if cocksucking is more work than fun, just give it up. Life is too short for a bad blow job."

As with all sex acts, there is no single "right way" to give a perfect hummer—as long as you put your mouth around his cock, you are on the right track. The best way to perfect your technique is to find out what feels good to your partner (by trial and error, and by asking questions) and go with that. However, to get you started, we offer a few guidelines and tips to follow that will put you on the fast track to being a great giver of head.

YOU GOTTA LOVE IT

If you're going to master the art of giving great head, you have to love what you are doing. A man can tell if you are down there grappling with his penis while simultaneously thinking of bills that need to be paid, big deadlines at work, or that sexy bartender at the club last night. That's just not hot. This isn't just another thing on your "to do" list. Bill, 62, tells us about his worst blow job: "It was a mechanical performance, and she obviously wasn't into it. We had had a few drinks and it was taking forever. She kept asking, 'Are you close? Because my jaw is tired.' Eventually, it started to hurt. I ejaculated, but with little pleasure."

Sucking your man to climax should be just as fun for you as for him. Lance, 35, tells us about his best blow job experience: "It was long and slow. She looked into my eyes throughout and really seemed to be enjoying it as much as I was." Our best advice? Unwrap his cock like it's a birthday gift. Nibble, suck, and lick it like it's the most delectable treat you've ever tasted. Get turned on by turning him on.

FELLATIO: 1887, from L. fellatus, pp. of fellare "to suck," from PIE base *dhe- (see *fecund*. The sexual partner performing fellatio is a fellator; if female, a fellatrice or fellatrix.

BLOW: "move air," O.E. *blawan* "make an air current, sound a wind instrument" (class VII strong verb; past tense *bleow*, pp. *blawen*), from P.Gmc. *blæ-anan* (cf. O.H.G.*blaen*), from PIE *bhle- "to swell, blow up" (cf. L. *flare* "to blow"). Slang "do fellatio on" sense is from 1933, as *blow (someone) off*, originally among prostitutes (*blowjob* first recorded 1961 in the sexual sense; as recently as 1953 it meant "a type of airplane").[19]

ASSUME THE POSITION

To give great head, both you and your guy should be comfortable. You may want to start with him standing, and you kneeling in front of him. This position is extremely sexy, especially if you put on some eyeliner and look up at him with your best dirty-girl smirk.

Or you can have him stand at the side of your bed while you lie on your stomach, side, or back. This gives either him or you easy access to your breasts and pussy and can be a fun way to double your pleasure. Standing can get tiring for him after about ten minutes. If your guy hasn't climaxed yet, have him lie back on the bed or sit on the couch. Ideally, to give full attention to his cock and balls, you should cozy up between his legs on your knees. If you're on the floor, don't forget to put a pillow under your knees so you don't get a nasty carpet burn.

Another well-known and loved position is 69. In this arrangement, you lie on top of your man with your mouth at cock level and your pussy in his face. Sometimes it can be hard for you to focus on your man with your legs straddled about his head, especially if he is gifted with tongue and toy. But on the plus side, it's quite a treat if you can manage to get him to ejaculate in this position while simultaneously enjoying an orgasm of your own.

A very comfortable position, and one that works best if you have a partner who takes a long time to orgasm via oral sex, is to have your partner lie on his side and then lie alongside him with your mouth slightly lower than his penis. You can prop your head up on a pillow or your elbow if it's more comfy. This position prevents neck strain, which in turn gives you a lot of endurance.

MAKE IT AN EVENT

Did you know that there is an unofficial holiday dedicated to giving blow jobs? Yes, indeed, since Boston radio personality Birdsey first mentioned the idea in 2002, March 14 has become known as Steak and BJ Day. It's an easy holiday to honor since all your guy wants is a full tummy and your lips around his favorite little buddy.

But you shouldn't want to reserve BJs for a once-a-year-treat. Even if you do it more frequently, good head cannot be rushed, so make every blow job an event for your guy. Get creative! Jonathan, a 37-year-old pilot, says of one his most memorable BJ experiences, "My wife surprised me by playing cowgirl and had me drop my drawers and put my hands up. She worked it for ten minutes. I could barely stand. It was the best blow job ever!"

This is your chance to spoil him and show him how much you care (and earn some frequent flyer miles to be cashed in later for your own oral pleasure). Plan to spend anywhere from ten to forty minutes simply enjoying his penis. Let him play with you if he wants, but keep the focus on him.

START WITH A TEASE

The first part of your BJ session should be about trying out new tricks and getting him turned on. The difference between you and a "professional" is that you actually want to spend time with your man's penis. Get to know the little guy and figure out what types of maneuvers he enjoys!

FOR STARTERS ▼

Kiss and lick all the way from his lips to his throat to his nipples to his stomach and around his pubic region, carefully avoiding his penis (indulge your inner temptress). Then open your mouth wide and slide his cock into your mouth, trying not to let your lips or tongue touch his shaft.

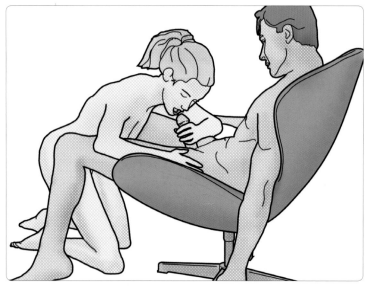

First, assume the position. It's important to be comfortable during a blow job.

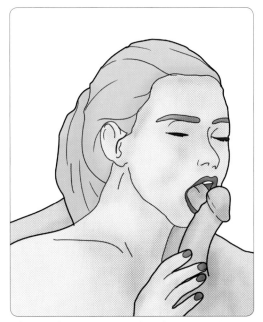 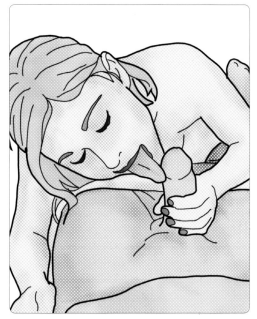

Stimulate his shaft and glans with a little tongue play.

Once you've enveloped the entirety of his cock (or as much as you are able), close your lips tightly and lick and suck on the up stroke. Open wide and repeat on the down stroke, creating an alternate teasing and sucking rhythm.

THE SLAP ▲ (LEFT)
Take his shaft and slap it gently against your cheeks, lips, and outstretched tongue while looking him in the eyes.

TONGUE PLAY ▲ (RIGHT)
Lick up and down the underside of his shaft and around his glans. Treat his cock like a lollipop and find out how many licks it takes to get to the center. With your mouth wrapped around the base of his cock, flick your tongue up and down the shaft while simultaneously creating a pulsing action with your lips (think of a sucker fish).

BALL HANDLING ▼

Nothing says "I love/lust/like you" more than some generous ball handling. These often-ignored body parts are full of sensation and should become a part of your sexual repertoire. Try kneeling in front of him, tilting your head back, and gripping one or both of his testicles between your lips. Suck them gently into your mouth and flick your tongue all around. If you have both balls in your mouth at once, be careful when you release them—if you are too abrupt they can knock against each other and cause a little pain. One ball at a time can be released a little more abruptly, but be gentle anyway. While sucking on his balls, reach up with your hand and stroke his cock to keep it nice and hard, or have him stroke his cock while you suckle his balls. Conversely, you may want to give his shaft all the attention it can handle with your mouth, while gently tugging down on his balls with your hands in a "milking" motion.

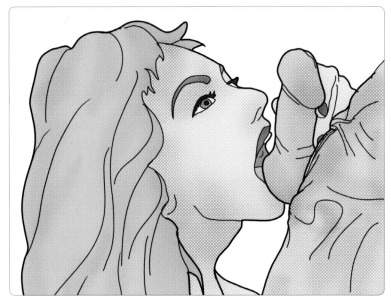

Draw his testicles into your mouth as you stimulate his shaft with your hand.

SPICE IT UP

Try chilling your tongue with ice cubes for a cool blow job. Or you can take a sip of hot tea or cider before wrapping your lips around his rod for a warming sensation. Try dipping him in chocolate sauce, honey, or whipped cream for a tasty treat. There is also a plethora of edible lubes and ointments that create all manner of tastes and sensations available at your local or online adult store. Just don't try slurping him with a mouthful of red wine or hot peppers; doing so can cause a painful burning along his urethra.

AURAL ORAL

Dirty talk is fun, and it doesn't have to be reserved for intercourse or phone sex. You can talk to your guy between licks and sucks and say naughty things like, "I'm so hungry for your cock. I can't wait to swallow all your cum." This will certainly push him closer to orgasm. Just don't say things like, "Honey, did you remember we're going to dinner at my parents' tomorrow night?" because that's not sex talk. That's just talk (and probably the reason cavemen invented blow jobs in the first place).

And of course, encourage him to dirty talk to you while your mouth is busy working his cock. It's fun to have him tug at your hair and call you his dirty little girl.

The classic hummer is also a great way to express yourself aurally. Push the tip of his penis to the back of your throat and hum him your favorite tune. The vibrations will send his penis a-tingling and possibly a-spilling.

Take his shaft as far into your mouth as possible, cup his balls in your hands and guide them gently toward your lower lip. While rubbing the tip of his cock on the roof of your mouth or in your throat, take your tongue and lower lip and lap at his balls. This will give your man the sensation of having two girls at once, but it's just you.

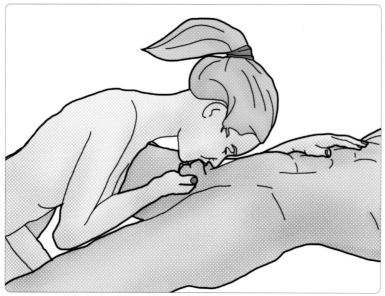

With his shaft all the way in your mouth, lap at his testicles with your lower lip or tongue.

WATCH THOSE TEETH!

The most common complaint we heard among men is that their partners are careless with their teeth. Remember: No matter how big or delicious it may be, his penis is not corn on the cob. Be careful with those teeth, ladies! When stroking a man from base to tip with your mouth, try covering your teeth with your lips. Describing a bad blow job, Lawrence says, "The woman had teeth like the Abominable Snowman creature in the old *Rudolph the Red-Nosed Reindeer* cartoon. She gave a whole new meaning to the phrase *severe head injuries*."

A little bit of teeth can be a good thing, though, when properly maneuvered. Some men actually love it when you give the shaft a little careful chewing—not too high around the head (the area around the base of the head can be particularly sensitive and is best left to the lips and tongue), but if you chew lower around the center of the shaft this can be a highly pleasurable sensation for your guy. Says Victor, 54, "The best blow job I ever had was when my wife lay on her back and turned her head to the side and I fucked her mouth and felt her lips, teeth, tongue, and the inside of her cheek. It was the mix of all those textures with each thrust." This gentle, toothy technique doesn't work for everyone, so try it and be sure to ask your man if he likes it; if not, switch up your method immediately. And whatever you do: DON'T BITE!

RHYTHM AND CONSISTENCY

Once you've teased him mercilessly and have him rock hard and ready to explode, it's time to bring him to climax, and this requires rhythm and consistency. Each man has his own favorite rhythm: Some like it hot and fast, some like it at a slower pace, some prefer a very strong grip, and some can get off with the touch of a feather. The key here is to find your man's preference, get into it, and keep at it until he reaches climax. Whatever you do, when you get into the rhythm, don't change anything—unless you want to prolong his ejaculation! For a foolproof way to keep up the momentum, set your iPod to a song with a steady beat and keep sucking him to the rhythm. For

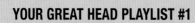

YOUR GREAT HEAD PLAYLIST #1
The tease: "Sexy" by Black Eyed Peas
Deep throat: "Ride Wit Me" by Nelly
The climax: "Candy Shop" by 50 Cent

YOUR GREAT HEAD PLAYLIST #2
The tease: "Crazy" Aerosmith
Deep throat: "Brick House" The Commodores
The climax: "Pour Some Sugar on Me" Def Leppard

the grand finale, it is very effective to use one or both hands (depending on how big he is and how much pressure he needs) to form a ring that grips around the base of his shaft. While stroking him with your hands, complete the sensation using your mouth on the upper half of his cock to keep it wet and slippery with your saliva (or add a couple drops of water-based lube). Stroke up and down in one long motion simultaneously using your hand and mouth. You can slip your hand over the tip of his penis as your mouth comes up (and practice saying something dirty). Tickle his head and the underside of his cock with your tongue as you stroke and suck him to a tasty climax.

DEEP THROAT

Although deep throat isn't a necessary trick to know, it is the one maneuver that separates good head from great head. Says Jose, 37, of his best blow job: "She was very hungry for my cock, and not many can deep throat me, but she did and she didn't stop until she had every bit of my cum on her tongue." Deep throat doesn't come naturally to everyone; some girls are a little more prone to gagging then others. But as with anything you try, practice makes perfect.

POSITION

Try a position where you can tilt your head up and create straight passage down your throat (think of how a sword-swallower looks when he prepares to ingest a 3-foot [0.9 m] sword). Examples of this are kneeling in front of your partner, lying alongside him so your head is slightly lower than his penis, or lying on your back so that your head hangs off the edge of the bed.

RELAX

While learning to perform deep throat, it's best if you are fully relaxed before starting. Take a nice, long, hot bath. Drink a glass of wine. Have your partner give you a long, sensual body massage—do whatever relaxes you the best. The more relaxed you are when you begin, the easier it will be to learn the deep-throat technique.

LUBRICATION

Lube is critical to excellent deep throat. An erect penis will slide much easier along the tongue and into the throat if it is well lubricated. Saliva works, but using a lubricant is longer-lasting and more effective. There are a variety of flavored and tasteless lubricants that can be used for oral pleasure at your local or online adult store. Another option (and porn-star secret) is the makeup remover called Albolene. It is nontoxic, odorless, and tasteless and can be purchased at any major drugstore.[20]

Although not necessary, an anesthetic can be useful in taming a particularly active gag reflex. Try spraying a topical anesthetic like Chloraseptic on the back of the tongue.

Dr. Dick says:

"Did you know that the gag response is least active in the morning? That's right, my pretties—you're gonna have to know things like this if you aspire to getting a gold medal in cocksucking. Besides, tidbits like this also make for the most charming dinner party trivia."

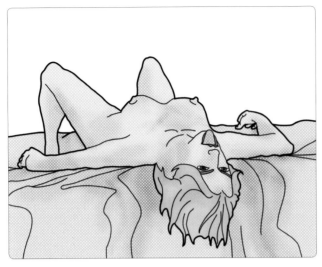

◀ To prepare for deep throat, lie with your head hanging off the bed and extend your tongue.

▼ Relax and draw your man's penis into the back of your throat.

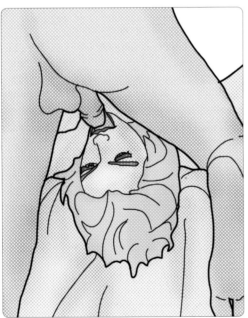

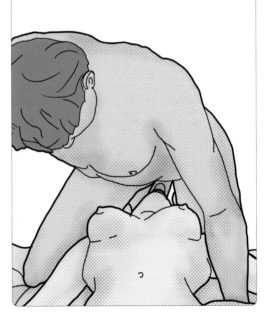

TECHNIQUE ◂

Once you're in position, slightly tilt your head back and extend the tip of your tongue just past your bottom lip. Flatten the back of your tongue and say "aaaah." Open your throat as you would if you were yawning. This will help to prevent the gag reflex from activating.

Take a deep breath and slowly slide the length of the penis into your mouth and along your tongue. When you feel the urge to gag, pause, take a deep breath through your nose, and hold the penis there as long as possible, then withdraw it. Repeat this process as many times as you can. Practice makes perfect!

When you get to the point where the head of his cock actually enters the throat, you may feel a little resistance. It will help to use your tongue to pull the penis in deeper. When you reach the point where you feel the gag reflex, pause for a moment, then, without removing the penis from your mouth, extend your tongue out a little farther and then pull your tongue back in your mouth, pulling the penis along with it.

THE HUMMER

Once you are practiced in the art of deep throat, try humming a tune when the head of your man's cock reaches the back of your throat. This creates an unbelievable vibrating sensation (yes, vibrations—he likes vibrations almost as much as you do).

Even if you aren't an expert deep-throat artist, your man will appreciate you for trying. Tell him you want to practice as much as possible, and do it!

TO SPIT OR TO SWALLOW?

Some women love the taste of semen, and others can't stand it. In our survey, 46 percent of the women said they enjoy the taste of semen, while 27 percent said they don't like it and 19 percent told us that they never taste the stuff. But connoisseurs may have noticed that not every man's cum tastes the same. In our discussions with women, we've discovered that the flavors can range in taste from fresh cucumbers, to Peanut M&Ms, to bitter coffee, and can even vary from day to day based on his diet and health.

Swallowing his cum is the cleanest finish to a blow job, and most men really appreciate it. But by no means is it necessary! If you really can't stand the idea of swallowing semen, it's also very exciting to have him squirt his juices all over your face or breasts (this is known as the "money shot" in adult films). This can be extremely visually stimulating for both you and your man and an ideal close to a perfect BJ. If you would rather take it in your mouth and spit it out, it's best to have a tissue readily available to spit into—otherwise you might give him the impression that you are "grossed out" by his cum. That's just not sexy and is potentially damaging to his male ego.

NUTRITION FACTS

"One teaspoon of semen contains 5 calories, 150 mg of protein, 11 mg of carbohydrates, 6 mg fat, 3 mg cholesterol, 7 percent U.S. RDA potassium and 3 percent U.S. RDA copper and zinc."[21]

—Johnson and Everitt, *Essential Reproduction* (2000)

If you do choose to swallow but don't want to taste it, you can either shoot it like you would an oyster or a shot of tequila, or you can push his cock to the back of your throat when he comes so that it's already past your taste buds. Not to worry if you swallow a shot of semen every day: It is not bad for you—and at only five calories a serving, it won't lead to weight gain.

ORAL SEX AND THE RISK OF INFECTIONS

Now just because you are an oral sex goddess doesn't mean you should go around practicing on just any man's cock. It's important to know your partner and his sexual history and health before engaging in any manner of unprotected sex, and this includes oral sex. Bill Clinton may have led us to believe that blow jobs are not sex, but in this context they most definitely are. There is a chance you can become infected with a whole cocktail of nasty STIs like chlamydia, HPV, gonorrhea, herpes, hepatitis, and others, including HIV (although cases of HIV infection via oral sex are rare or insufficiently documented).[22] The existence of wounds or lesions on his genitals or in your mouth significantly increases your risk of becoming infected. If you insist on slipping your lips around a random hot guy's pole, you definitely will want to get some flavored condoms and wrap it up.

CUM COMES IN MANY FLAVORS

Although most women reported that semen tastes slightly salty, others shared a wider variety of flavor experiences, including honey, cream, coconut, bananas, oranges, sugar, pineapple, bread, pudding, liquid sunflower seeds, satay sauce, salty fries, olives, celery, cake frosting, sushi, chocolate-covered pretzels, salt water taffy, vanilla ice cream, rice, mushrooms, asparagus, egg whites, grapefruit, yogurt, salsa, lemon, romaine lettuce, tea, Fritos, anchovies, wallpaper paste, oysters, cookies, popcorn, a Big Mac, and beer.

HOW TO GIVE A HEART-STOPPING HAND JOB

THE HAND JOB has been an integral part of the human sexual condition probably for as long as humans have had hands—yet another reason to applaud the evolutionary triumph that is the opposable thumb. Proof that men love hand jobs can be found in places from as long ago as an erotic painting of a hand job immortalized on a brothel wall in Ancient Roman Pompeii, to modern day promises of "happy endings" at massage parlors.

Indeed, one could make the argument that the typical man's penis will spend significantly more time in the embrace of a palm (whether it be his own or another's) than it will in the warm, wet confines of a mouth, vagina, or other orifice. However, the common meeting of hand and cock does not make it a ho-hum sex act.

Three major obstacles usually stand in the way of a woman pursuing the art of giving a great hand job.

OBSTACLE #1:
HE KNOWS HIS EQUIPMENT BETTER THAN YOU EVER WILL

The first obstacle women encounter is the fact that men have already had years of practice with manual stimulation. After all, it is the only sex act that a typical man can perform on himself (hence *master*bation)—unless he's extraordinarily flexible like James (played by Paul Dawson) from the 2006 film *Shortbus*, who was able to auto-fellate himself. This sets the standard for hand jobs pretty high and may leave you wondering how you can compete with (and gain mastery over) what a man knows how to do best.

Take heart. It seems that most men are actually hardwired to prefer hand jobs to a good masturbation session. Says Jim, a 34-year-old engineer, "I don't know what it is, but my girlfriend's hand feels so much better on my cock than my own does. It's like her hand is electric!" The reason for this "electric" current could be that men produce significantly higher levels of testosterone—the predominant male sex hormone—when being touched by another than they do when touching themselves.[23]

If you're afraid your phalangeal talents might not be up to par with his, give yourself a little pep talk, keeping these things in mind:

- Man is a visual creature, and seeing your hand—with its delicate, slim fingers and sexy, manicured nails—wrapped around his hard shaft is a hell of a lot more stimulating than seeing his own beefy digits strokin' the pole. Taylor, a 38-year-old bartender, says, "Doing anything with someone else is *always* better than doing it alone, and that includes hand-on-cock action."

- You can do things at certain angles with your two hands that he simply cannot do. "The best HJ is two-handed, with twisting and a lot of lube. If her hand is on the head of my penis when I orgasm, it literally feels so good it hurts," says A.J., 35.

- He's been yanking his own chain since he was a pup and probably does it the same way time after time. Your creative manhandling will bring him new sensations that are sure to cream his Popsicle. Dan, a 30-something Web designer says, "The best hand job for me is long, gentle, drawn out, teasing . . . the opposite of the way I'd do it myself."

- Often, when performing a hand job, context is everything. Says Jimmy, a 30-something executive, "The best hand job I've ever had was the first one given to me by a person who wasn't me. Everything happened inside my trousers while in her mother's living room with her parents asleep upstairs. Stylistically maybe it wasn't the best ever, but the enormity of the event will mean it's always the *best*."

OBSTACLE #2:
HAND JOBS ARE A POOR COUSIN TO BLOW JOBS AND INTERCOURSE

The second obstacle that keeps a woman from embarking on the great hand job quest is simple: She's great at giving blow jobs, and she finds the hand job to be its less glamorous counterpart. Indeed, for some men, a hand job really isn't high up on the list of exciting sexual scenarios. As 28-year-old Luke puts it, "A hand job to me is a waste of time. I can always do them better myself. It's like putting a box of shredded wheat in front of me when I know she's hiding a box of donuts in her skirt. I want the donuts!"

However, there are times when only a hand job will do. One of the beautiful qualities of the hand job is that it lends itself more easily than other sex acts to a wider variety of settings and situations. Says Dave, a 40-something doctor, "The best I've ever had was in an airport parking lot, with folks going back and forth pretty much constantly. The excitement that we might get caught with her hand on my cock was all I needed."

Another thing to keep in mind is that you may find yourself with a man who actually prefers the hand job to the blow job. (It's okay ladies. You can pick your jaw up off the floor now.) For these reasons, it's important for you to take up the challenge and learn the skills to wow your guy right out of his pants.

If you're a deep-throat enthusiast, keep in mind that a hand job is better than a blow job when:

- You're having dinner with his parents but you need him to come . . . *now*! Think of the oddly sexy scene from *The Wedding Crashers* (2005) in which Gloria Cleary (Isla Fisher) manually has her way with Jeremy Grey (Vince Vaughn) at the family dinner table. Discreet hand-under-the-table action will go over much better than spending an inordinate amount of time under the table looking for that dropped napkin.

- You want to practice the art of dirty talk while you get him off. Your sexy vocal ministration just doesn't sound quite the same when slurred through a mouthful of his member. Refer to chapter 6, "Sexy Secret Spots Off the Cock," for ideas on the art of dirty talk.
- You want to use your mouth for other things, like lapping at a nipple, biting his neck, or licking his butthole.

OBSTACLE #3:

I NEED TO BE ABLE TO CRUSH GRAPEFRUITS WITH A SINGLE SQUEEZE

The third obstacle to becoming a great giver of hand pleasure is specific to that class of women who despise bowling. If you are the type of woman who finds the first couple minutes of bowling to be okay (despite the hideous shoes), but then realizes it becomes tedious and exhausting because it hurts your hands, you are probably well aware of this obstacle.

So what's a girl to do if her hand cramps up after a few minutes of wanking his willy? Before you spend your free time manually crushing walnuts to strengthen the thenar muscles in your thumbs, try the following:

1. **Change it up.** Keep in mind that for the first several minutes of your hand job, the goal is to get him warmed up and extremely aroused so that he can enjoy an earth-shattering orgasm. So don't start off with the repetitive stroking motions that will eventually cause his climax. Try a variety of techniques (explained later in this chapter) to get your hands warmed up for the inevitable explosion. Hopefully, by the time you get to those tiring repetitive motions, it will only take a few strokes before he comes.

2. **Remember: You have two hands for a reason.** When one gets tired, it's time to call for backup. You can alternate between hands so neither one reaches full fatigue before the climax. However, when switching hands, it's important not to lose your rhythm as he approaches ejaculation—if you do, it will prolong his pleasure and lead to more work for your hands.

3. **Use different positioning.** It can be much more exhausting to perform a hand job while kneeling between his legs. Try lying beside him and massaging his member while resting your forearm on his thigh. This position also offers a great level of intimacy because you can kiss his lips, ears, and neck as you play.

4. Cheat a little. Although a hand job can't *technically* be considered a hand job without a happy ending, this doesn't mean that you are obligated to finish him up manually. When the hands can go no further you can bring in a toy, your mouth, or (if you are sufficiently aroused) just hop on top to finish him off.

For those of you who are ready to whip out your bowling glove and embrace the age-old art of finger-to-frenulum action, let's lube up and move on!

HAND JOB RECON:
GATHER INFORMATION BEFORE YOU PULL HIS POLE

According to information from the Kinsey Institute, a study done in 2002 of undergraduate college students found that 98 percent of men (and 44 percent of women) claimed to have ever masturbated. So unless your guy is part of that freakish two percent who claimed to never have enjoyed the art of self-pleasure, chances are your man has spent years developing a unique and specific touch to get off. Your first assignment is to get him to show you just how he does it. Watching a man stroke himself can be incredibly sexy, and your partner will most likely thrill in demonstrating his dexterity for you. However, ask him to do so in an alluring and sexy way; he probably won't want to jack off for you if you make your request between sips of coffee while reading the paper.

If your guy is shy but you want him to show you how to play with his penis, here are a few suggestions:

- Surprise him by joining him during his morning shower. Take his hand in yours, encircle both around his cock, and ask him to show you what he likes. The higher testosterone levels in his body, induced by your touch, will make him a more able and willing participant in this activity, and the silky suds will ensure there's enough lube if he needs or likes it. We promise he won't be able to refuse your sweet request as you stand before him nude, batting your eyelashes, and seductively biting your lip.
- Tell him you'll give him a show if he gives you one. For reconnaissance purposes, you won't want to masturbate simultaneously—after all, you'll want your senses about you to pay attention to his technique. Masturbating for him first should get him in the proper mood.

- At the end of the day, cuddle up with him in bed and playfully ask him to use your hand with his. If the lights are out, he may feel more comfortable to truly let loose and enjoy, and if your hand is part of the action, you'll get a good sense of his preferred pressures and speeds.

Take notes! Mental notes, that is, unless you think your guy would enjoy a scientist–subject role-playing session. Men can go from situation normal to orgasm rather quickly, especially when going it solo (they've perfected the process, remember), so you'll want to observe a few things in particular. If you've convinced your guy to be your willing subject, it's time to closely observe:

- Pay attention to what kind of stroke he begins with. Is it slower and softer? Or does he go into it full-throttle? Does his hand circle his testicles at all? Does it play with the tip? How he begins to self-stimulate will give you good ideas for what he might like when you begin the arousal phase of your hand job.

INTERESTING NOTES ON MALE MASTURBATION

Men do indeed enjoy their solo time. In the O&C survey, 25 percent of men admitted to masturbating one to three times per week, 17 percent said they did it every other day, and 24 percent said they do it every day. And 43 percent of these said it only takes them two to five minutes to reach ejaculation.

Some of the more colorful places men like to pleasure themselves include:

- "Alone in the den."

- "On the deck behind my house."

- "In my car."

- "On the patio under the heater."

- "In a laundry room. I used to raid dryers and masturbate on girls' panties. The sexier, the better."

- "Outside in the woods."

- "In front of the computer." (Surprise, surprise!)

- And ladies, 51 percent of men admitted to having masturbated at work at least once!

- When you hear his breathing quicken, observe how his stroking changes. It is probably a faster movement, and his hand is likely applying more pressure. This is the build-up that will get him closer to climax. Pay attention to the length of his strokes. Are they focused on the head of his shaft, or do they run the entire length of his cock? Does he apply more pressure on the down stroke, the up stroke, or do they appear to be even?
- As his breathing increases and he appears to be close to climax, again take special note of the stroke and pressure he is using. This will serve as a baseline for you; consider it the "go to" move when you're ready to wrap up the work of art that will be your hand job and bring him to climax. He could be applying what looks to be an alarming amount of strength and pressure, or he could be using a feather-touch. This "go to" stroke will most likely not waver as he shoots his wad.

As you survey the way that your lover loves himself, keep in mind that you're not going to exactly replicate his masturbatory habits. Changing the "hand script" and trying new moves will lengthen your playtime and increase his pleasure. But by watching and understanding his techniques, you'll know where to go if you need to reset your efforts at any time, and you'll know just what stroke to use when it's time for the grand finale.

HAND JOB TECHNIQUES THAT EVERY WOMAN NEEDS TO KNOW

Now it's time to take matters into your own hands. Here are the quintessential techniques gleaned from hands-on hand job research. As you spend more time with cock in hand, be sure to try one or more of these during each session. New stimulation and manipulation will only make your hand jobs more exciting and enjoyable for him. Don't be afraid to check in with him as you try new maneuvers. And remember: Lube is your friend for all of these!

THE BASIC STROKE

Also known as "milking the penis," this is the most important stroke to learn because, for the majority of men, the basic stroke is one and the same as the "go to" stroke mentioned earlier. Slide one or both hands up and down his entire shaft. Speed and pressure vary.

The basic stroke can be used in conjunction with perineum and ball massage. To add to the "milking" sensation, gently tug down on his balls with one hand while stroking his penis with the other.

The basic stroke has a few variations. Use your recon data and experiment with his cock to determine which works best for your guy. He may prefer one of the following strokes to the others, or he may enjoy all of them:

- Try using only your forefinger and thumb connected in a ring to apply pressure. In this variation, you don't touch his penis with your palm or other fingers.

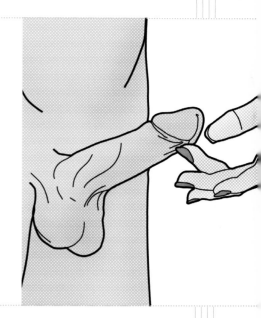

 A TIP FOR THE TIP (OR HOW TO FINGER HIS FRENULUM)

The frenulum is the most sensitive part of his cock because it contains a large concentration of nerve endings. It is located on the underside of the penis where the ridge of the head meets the rest of the shaft. Tickle or massage this spot with one hand while stroking the rest of his cock with the other and you will have him moaning for more. Another great technique for stimulating the frenulum is to create a circle with your thumb and forefinger and stroke up and down, applying more pressure as you go over the cock ridge.

- Use your forefinger and thumb as the main stroking mechanism, while the rest of your fingers apply only light, tickling pressure. This technique combines the firm touch of forefinger and thumb with the feathery sensation created by the rest of the fingers.
- Combine the pressure of your fingers and your entire palm in a uniform, firm caress.

How do you determine which variation of the basic stroke your lover likes best? Just ask him, of course!

THE SHIMMY ▼
Use both palms and rub the shaft between them, shimmying up and down his length. This technique calls for very gentle pressure and plenty of lube.

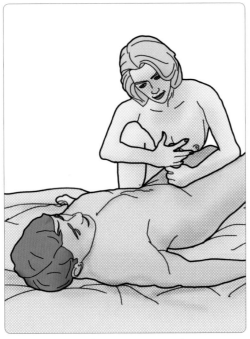

Give his penis the shimmy and rub the shaft between both your hands.

THE TWIST ▶
Encircle his cock with both hands (or the ol' forefinger–thumb ring) and twist up and down his length. A variation is to use one hand to do the twist while the other massages the frenulum and cock head. When making any twisting motion, use gentle pressure and lots of lube.

THE BREAST STROKE
When he's on his back, let his cock rest against his stomach. In a smooth, upward motion, use one or both palms to skim over his testicles and up the underside of his shaft. For added stimulation, allow your breasts to tickle up his cock after your palms. This provides a great visual for him, as well.

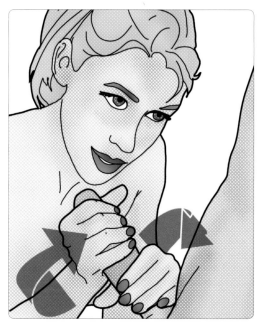

With lubed up hands, twist up and down his length.

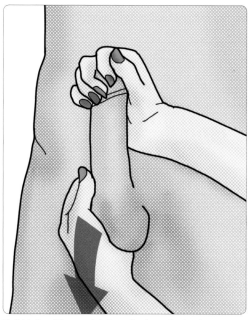

Roll his head in your lubricated palm to "palm the knob" while you gently tug down on his scrotum.

THE TEASE

If you want to add a little bit of tantalizing torture to your hand job, and perhaps slow him down, stroke and play with his shaft with absolutely no touch to the cock head. If done right, you'll have him thrusting in your hands. Be sure to give him your best bad-girl look to let him know that you know exactly what you're doing.

PALM THE KNOB ▲

On the flip side, try ignoring his shaft. Simply roll his cock head in your well-lubricated, cupped palm. Use both clockwise and counterclockwise rotations. Wax on, wax off!

THE NEVER-ENDING THRUST

Encircle one hand (say, the right) around the head of his penis and slide it all the way down to the base. Before your right hand leaves the base of his cock, begin the same motion with your left hand. Some men say this technique feels like a never-ending thrust into orgasmic bliss. Change directions for a different sensation.

BLOW HIS MIND . . . AND HIS HEAD

This one is not for the faint of heart or the anally shy, but perfect for when your man is fresh out of the shower. After you've turned him on and tuned him up, have him get on all fours and climb up behind him. Reach around with one hand and use the basic stroke to milk his cock while you run your tongue along his perineum and anus. This position can be incredibly vulnerable for a man and, if done right, will literally have him shaking on his knees.

SLOW HIM DOWN

If you see your man escalating faster than you would like and you have a few more techniques you still want to try out, squeeze the base of his penis with your thumb and forefinger until his breathing slows. This will cut off some of the blood flow to his cock and will stem the ejaculatory process—at least momentarily.

USING PERFECT PRESSURE

Let us pontificate on pressure. Many women use less pressure and vigor than they should because they fear hurting their men. Don't be afraid to use a firm hand (especially if you're using lubricant). You'd be surprised at how much pressure most men enjoy.

But you don't want to use *too* much pressure (especially without adequate lubrication). Several men we surveyed complained that they suffered from friction burn as a result of overzealous penis pumping. Says Mark, a 30-something consultant, "One girl I was with seemed to have the unconquerable urge to grip only from halfway down the shaft to the bottom and, at the same time, pull down with all the strength she could muster. How my foreskin never became detached from the head of my cock I'll never know!"

Not to worry. A well-timed "Do you like this?" or "Do you want it harder or softer?" will steer you in the right direction (not to mention if you've done your recon mission, you'll have a clear idea of how he likes it). We guarantee that once you have a good grasp of what kind of pressure your man prefers, applying it will feel like sexy second nature to you. You'll be able to stop worrying about whether you're doing it too hard or soft, and you can move on to learning and practicing more varied techniques.

LUBE IS YOUR ALLY

Even if he doesn't use lube while masturbating, you should always use it when you give him a hand job (unless, of course, he instructs you otherwise). Men love to put their penises in warm, wet places (à la *American Pie*). Lubricant helps you create this delicious effect, minus the cinnamon and nutmeg, and protects against chafing and friction burn.

Among the men in our survey, a common complaint regarding less-than-satisfactory hand jobs referred to women not using enough lubrication or having rough or chapped hands. Conversely, many men who described excellent hand jobs made mention of the woman's soft skin and the fact that she used plenty of lubrication. The lesson: Lube him up and be sure to keep your mitts moisturized.

For important information on what type of lube you should use for manual play, refer to chapter 7, "Toys for Boys."

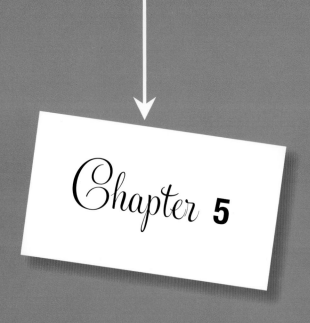

Chapter 5

FUNKY BUTT LOVIN' AND THE P-SPOT

APPROACHING ANAL PLAY, especially with straight men, is something akin to knocking on the gates of the forbidden kingdom. You may find that your lover has never had anyone touch him "there," let alone lick or penetrate it with finger or toy. However, if you learn how to excel in the anal arts, you will be able to provide him with a unique pleasure that no other erotic touch or technique can provide.

Of course, as with anything else, straight men's attitudes about anal play (on themselves, mind you) vary greatly. Some men are absolute anal fanatics, like Jake, a 32-year-old insurance agent, who says, "There's absolutely nothing like a finger in the ass during an orgasm!"

For other men, bringing up anal play may inspire the silent treatment: With butt cheeks clenched, they may just give you the cold, stony, "How could you?" glare. And still others may get downright squeamish: "You want to touch me, *wherrrre?*" (Imagine a high-pitched, whiny-little-girl voice coming out of your manly man.) If in no other area than this one, the key is to proceed with tenderness and respect.

ANATOMY OF HIS ANUS

Ladies, let's get down to the brass tacks of how to anally pleasure your man. Remember the song "Dem Dry Bones"?

> *The knee bone's connected to the thigh bone.*
> *The thigh bone's connected to the hip bone.*
> *The hip bone's connected to the back bone.*
> *Oh hear the word of the Lord!*

Let's fill in the missing blanks:

> *The scrotum's connected to the perineum.*
> *The perineum's connected to the butthole.*
> *The butthole's connected to the anal canal.*
> *The canal cozies up to the seminal vesicle.*
> *The vesicle's connected to the prostate.*
> *The prostate's connected to . . . pleasure.*
> *Oh, hear the word of the Lord!*

The lesson? If you know this area and know what to do with the anus and prostate, some subtle additions can take his orgasm from "Heck yeah!" to "Hallelujah!"

THE PERTY PERINEUM ▼

Pretend your forefinger is oh-so-lightly taking a tour of your lover's body. From the most obvious focal point, his penis, trace lightly over his testicles to the tissue just below that connects to the anus. This tissue is called the perineum. Other words for this tissue include *tweener* (as in, it's 'tween the balls and the ass) and *taint* (it ain't the testicles, and it ain't the ass). Don't let these slang terms misguide you; this area is not to be passed over. Though it's a small region, the perineum has a large number of nerve endings, which means that manipulation of this area is greatly pleasurable for him. Try lightly licking it, tickling it with your fingertips, or massaging it in circular motions—this will have the added benefit of stimulating his prostate from outside his body.

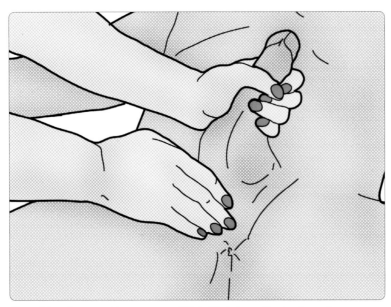

Caress his perineum and the area around his butthole in gentle, circular motions.

THE BEAUTIFUL BUTTHOLE

From the perineum, let your finger slide down to his anus. That lovely, puckering protuberance is literally bursting with nerve endings. Lick it, press it, massage it with love—doing any of these will bring a delectable pleasure to your sex play. Most men won't orgasm by anal stimulation alone, but the pleasure it lends adds a whole new dimension to sex. As Charles, 56, a magazine editor, says, "There are few perfections in this world like it."

Use anal stimulation to kick your foreplay up a notch. And if used simultaneously with a blow job, hand job, or intercourse, you'll truly give him an orgasm to remember.

THE INTIMACY INSIDE THE RECTUM ▼

Now, with lots of lube and the utmost permission, pass your finger through the anus into the rectum. If your lover is aroused, he should experience no pain because the sphincter should open

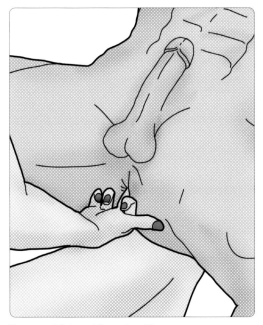 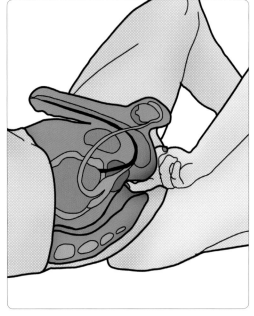

Ease your lubricated finger into his rectum.

easily to you. It's a slow, gentle process, but if and when your finger makes it inside, take your time and play a little. Some men enjoy subtle in-out action, while others prefer a constant pressure. Be sure to check in with him and remember his vulnerability here—after all, you are the penetrator now. If you do finger-fuck him to climax (this is usually done in tandem with penile stimulation), you'll actually feel his anus pulse around your finger. A heady experience, indeed!

A NOTE ON PERMISSION

When it comes to sex, we usually think that permission is something we must give to men, or that it's something they should try to obtain from us. We live in a cock-centric society where it is often assumed that if he's hard, it's okay for a gal to climb aboard. In other words, when it comes to sex, permission isn't a two-way street.

CODE OF CONDUCT FOR PLEASURING HIS BUNGHOLE (WE MEAN THE ONE IN HIS ASS, NOT IN HIS WINE CASK)

- Always cut and file your fingernails so there are no sharp edges to snag or hurt him.
- If you use toys, make sure you file off on any rough edges of plastic that could hurt him.
- Anal play should never hurt, so if you inflict pain (and he isn't asking for it), back off.
- Always use a good-quality, water- or silicone-based lube, and plenty of it.
- Be gentle, go slow, and move forward only with permission!

"Regarding negotiating consent, we assume that women don't have to. As women, we don't learn to ask what men really want and we don't have to deal with the implications of him saying no," says Dr. Glenda. "By not having to negotiate consent, we are not owning what we want as women, nor are we granting him the full range of being a complete sexual partner."

If we learn how to ask permission and communicate with our man here, at the threshold of the "back door," perhaps it will open other doors, so to speak, and we can learn to negotiate consent for every sexual act as well-rounded lovers and partners.

THE PERFECT PROSTATE

If you're both open to further exploration, move your finger into his anal canal, with the pad turned toward the upper side (toward the belly). When you go deep enough to lose a knuckle, or about an inch (2.54 cm) in, you will find a bump of tissue about the size of a walnut. You've hit gold: the prostate.

The prostate is the gland that surrounds the neck of the bladder and urethra (the tube that carries urine from the bladder and delivers semen and seminal fluid during orgasm). The prostate is partly muscular and partly glandular, and as a sexual organ, the prostate secretes a slightly alkaline fluid that makes up 25 percent to 30 percent of semen (the rest of it is made up of spermatozoa and seminal vesicle fluid.) The alkalinity of the prostate fluid helps neutralize the acidity of the vaginal tract, which prolongs the lifespan of the sperm (the better to impregnate you with, my dear!). During orgasm, the prostate helps propel the fluid into the urethra.

Why does touching his prostate feel so damn good to him? It's a highly sensory organ with a large amount of nerve endings, and knowing how to touch and massage it will take his orgasm to a whole new level.

HOW TO PET THE PROSTATE ▼

It took only one silly scene in an even sillier movie for us to understand the raw power of the prostate massage. *Road Trip* (2000) features the character E.L. (played by Seann William Scott), who bends over and quickly comes in a cup thanks to the perfunctory manual manipulations of a prostate-milking nurse. As we heard her glove snap and watched his O face on the screen, we had to wonder, *Is it really possible to have a man melt (or come) in your hands like that?* Right then, we knew we had to learn it: the prostate massage.

For the perfect technique, we turned to the ultimate source, Dr. Dick.

Before you even start your sex play, have your man relax. Encourage him to take a hot shower, a warm bath, or try some deep breathing exercises. Make sure you've followed the code of conduct for anal play, have a ready supply of water- or silicone-based lube handy, and for goodness' sake, file your fingernails!

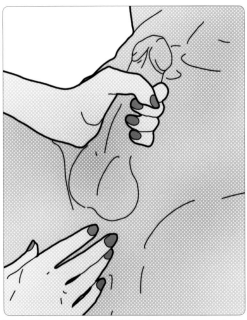
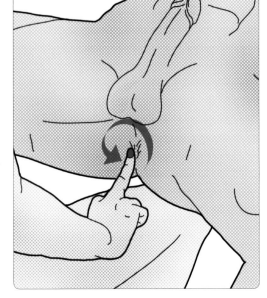

Warm him up by massaging his perineum and butthole.

The recommended position from which to start is to have your lover lie on his back so that you can sit between his legs. This gives you perfect access to the trifecta—his cock, balls, and anus. Next . . .

- Caress his dick with your lubed hand to get him to his happy place.
- Gradually slather some of that lube onto his balls and taint. While his legs are open, find his hole and play with his rosebud. Gently massage the area around his asshole, but don't slide your fingers in just yet. Simply let him get used to the feelings at the opening of his ass.
- Eventually, press the tip of your finger into his ass. If you do this while you're stroking his cock, you will find that his hole will actually open and invite your finger.
- Once he's comfortable with your fingertip inside, try pushing it in farther and moving it around a little. Then push it in and pull it out of his ass (think of it as finger-fucking your man).

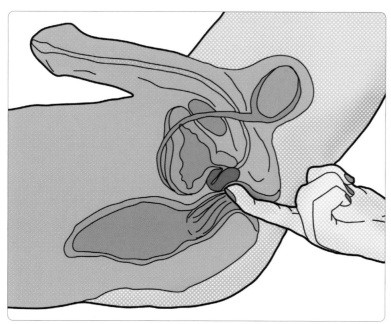

Gently press your finger into his rectum and locate his prostate.

- About an inch (2.54 cm) or so inside your man's ass, press your finger upward toward his navel, along the wall of his rectum. You'll discover the round bulb of tissue. It shouldn't be hard to find, particularly if your man is all horned up. It will feel smooth and hard, like a flat stone.
- Give that puppy a nice, gentle massage with your fingertip. If you're still stroking his wood, don't be surprised if this prostate massage gets him off. In fact, you will find that his prostate actually enlarges a bit and becomes firmer just as he is about to shoot. As he comes, you will also notice that his sphincter muscle will tighten around your finger and pulsate with each squirt.

And voila, ladies! You've performed a glorious prostate massage! You know what they say, now: Practice makes perfect.

SOME TECHNICAL TERMS

- **RIMMING:** Also known as analingus, this is the act of licking your lover's asshole. The tongue does not need to go inside.

- **PEGGING:** When a woman wears a strap-on dildo and penetrates her male lover's anus. This term came into widespread use after 2001 when it won over the terms *bob* and *punt* in a reader vote hosted by Dan Savage's "Savage Love" sex advice column.[24]

- **ANAL FISTING:** The act of putting an entire hand into the rectum. Usually the fingers are held loosely straight, in a beaklike shape, to get into the rectum, then followed by the rest of the hand. We said it before, and we'll say it again here: If you try this, use copious amounts of lubrication.

POSSIBLE ROADBLOCKS TO UTMOST ANAL PLEASURE

You may have a guy whose list of concerns about you playing between his butt cheeks is about as lengthy as the contract for your home mortgage. Let's discuss some of the roadblocks you could encounter (whether conscious or otherwise).

HIS COCK-CENTRIC NATURE

Many men (and some women) believe that the penis is the be-all, end-all of a man's sexual experience and pleasure. If your lover is one of these cock-centered types, he may balk at the suggestion that anal play can be incredibly arousing and sexual. After all, if you can easily get him off by pleasuring his pole, why even bother with all that other stuff? It will take some artful maneuvering with your stud to convince him that sex and pleasure are connected to so many more body parts and not just the genitals!

ANAL PLAY IS GAY!

As we discuss in chapter 9, "His Brain on Sex," many of the hang-ups surrounding anal play come from warped societal attitudes regarding homosexuality. Indeed, 36 percent of women we surveyed said they have been with a man who had problems with anal play being done on him. Says Terri, a 40-year-old software developer, "My current lover says no way. It's just not his deal, though I've told him he would like it. He licks me and anally fucks me, so I kind of think the issue isn't about pleasure for him."

Several other women simply report: "He thinks it would make him gay."

If your lover is reluctant because he thinks ass play is gay, remind him that that would only be true if gay men were the only ones with prostates.

OTHER AVERSIONS TO THE ASS

Survey says: Sixty-one percent of the men we surveyed said they enjoy anal stimulation, 15 percent said they do not, and 24 percent said they have never tried it. Reported negative aversions to anal stimulation (other than homophobic fears) include:

- "Not safe . . . two words: shigella and E. coli."
- "It's kinda boring."
- "Exterior stimulation is okay, but I'm uncomfortable with insertion. I always associate the sensation with enemas, which I feared and despised as a child."
- "A finger up the ass with a long fingernail is very uncomfortable."
- "I think it would really gross her out to touch my anus. But I would clean really well if I knew it were going to happen."

As you can see from this sample of comments, there are plenty of personal reasons that a man might shy away from a woman touching his derriere.

Men who actually enjoy anal play with their partners may give us even more insight into why his ass can seem so off-limits. Brandon, a 43-year-old loan officer, says, "Anal sex is one of many ways to express appreciation, care, love, and trust in one another." Similarly, Dave, a pharmaceutical rep, 31, confesses, "It's very forbidden, extremely sensitive and sexual, and I love the submissive aspect." For these men, indulging in anal play with their partners is an act of intimacy, trust, and submission. In other words, ladies, this is the one area where the man becomes the penetratee (of tongue, finger, toy, or fist) rather than the penetrator. If a man doesn't trust you or feel intimate with you, he may not feel comfortable submitting that part of his body to you.

MOVING PAST THE ROADBLOCKS: TENDERNESS AND RESPECT

We could just as well head this section with the two classic songs, Otis Redding's "Respect" and Chris Brown's "Try a Little Tenderness," because these are the two key elements you should always keep in mind and at heart when approaching a man's nether regions. Chances are, your lover will have at least one, if not all of the mental roadblocks we've discussed, and it is for these reasons that a woman needs to be at her gentlest when treading on his hallowed ground.

So how to proceed? Dr. Jenni recommends exploring the many different erogenous zones of your lover's body, not only the anal area. "I wouldn't push the anal thing too early; I might start with sensate focus on other areas of the body and then move toward less vanilla zones if it feels right." As you explore these sensitive areas, you may slowly convince your lover that his penis isn't his only possible source of pleasure, and this realization might make him more open to receiving anal stimulation.

Other steps include allowing him to play with you anally and sharing other sources of information with him regarding hetero enjoyment of anal play. If he reads an article about another straight man enjoying a strap-on, he may feel more comfortable with the idea himself.

Dr. Dick says:

"The best thing a woman can do is watch some hot butt-sex porn with her man, where the dude is on the receiving end of things. These are called pegging vids. There are also 'how to' videos such as *Tristan Taormino's Expert Guide to Anal Pleasure for Men.*"

THE BOTTOM LINE ON HIS BOTTOM IS "NO"

As Dr. Glenda reminds us, "Some men just aren't going to enjoy it. For them, it's 'Exit only, dude.'" Just as we're sure you have things you just don't or won't do in your sex life, there are men who will simply never enjoy anal play. If you have one of these men in your life, don't push it. Part of being a truly excellent lover is respecting your partner's boundaries.

KEEPING IT SAFE

TOY SAFETY

First, ladies, it's important to understand that the anal canal is not like the vagina. With the very narrow cervix that leads to the uterus, the vagina is, for the most part, a closed space. Not so with the anal cavity, colon, and lower intestine. This is one back door that also has a back door. When putting things up his butt, remember that there are several feet of organ in there, and if the object doesn't have a string or handle you can pull on or isn't anchored by a flared base, the two of you could be making a very embarrassing trip to the emergency room.

Dr. Glenda says:

"There's a whole world of physics that women and most straight men just don't get. There's no wall there, and there can be a vacuum effect when a person sticks objects up the ass. It's the straight boys who get overenthusiastic with anal play and end up at the doctor's. Gay boys tend to know their physical limits."

FECAL MATTER MATTERS

Anal play is always more fun for everyone when the "ick" factor has been removed. This means making sure he's freshly showered and clean. Usually, the best way to achieve this is to pop into the shower with him. If you do the job yourself, you'll know it's done to your standards of cleanliness—and soap makes a very nice lube!

In addition, keep in mind that the anal canal, which is just inside the rectum, is not a storage area for poo; it's just a passageway from the lower intestine. So if he has washed and you want to insert a finger, you won't encounter a nasty surprise.

Fecal matter is made up of about 75 percent water and a lot of bacteria. This means that, unlike urine, it is not sterile! Diseases like cholera, typhus, giardia, and hepatitis A can be contracted from accidental ingestion of feces. Obviously, this means it's extra important that you only tongue a squeaky-clean playground.

As a double precaution, have him evacuate up to a couple of hours before your anal play. And if you two are very serious about analingus, consider giving him an enema. (The doctor is in!) To practice truly safe sex, you can use a dental dam (or even plastic wrap) to create a thin barrier between your finger/tongue and his anus.

STI RISKS

Yes, anal play on him is a sexual activity and therefore brings the risk of sexually transmitted infection (STI). Sharing toys between his ass and your vagina, mouth, or ass can transmit any number of STIs. Herpes and HPV are transmitted via skin-to-skin contact, thus finger-fucking and fisting will put you at risk if you are not conscientious and clean about it. And any STIs that can be spread by giving him a nice juicy blow job can likewise be transmitted during analingus. These include syphilis, HPV, chlamydia, gonorrhea (with the possible risks of hepatitis B and HIV). Moreover, if you have herpes 1, the virus that causes mouth sores, you can give this to your lover during a rim job, especially if you have an active sore at the time. This will manifest as anal sores for him.

The important thing to remember, ladies, is to treat anal sex play just as you would any other sex play. Keep informed and use safer sex practices.

Chapter 6

SEXY SECRET SPOTS OFF THE COCK

THERE SEEMS TO BE a resounding message in response to common attitudes about heterosexual sex: It's not all about a hard cock! Men are detrimentally taught that sex, pleasure, orgasm (both his and hers), and everything in between are intrinsically linked to a long, hard, raging boner. All of the experts agree, from Paul Joannides, who writes, "Our society teaches us that sexual pleasure between a man and a woman depends on the man's ability to get hard and stay hard,"[25] to Dr. Ian Kerner, who says, "For most men, sex begins and ends with the penis and rarely extends beyond it."[26]

You may put too much stock in the almighty cock as well. (After all, they are pleasurable little playthings.) However, we encourage you to view the male body, and thus the male sexual experience, as something both broad and full of nuance. If you approach your lover as a whole person and body, not just a single appendage, sex will be much better for both of you. Here's a road map to some of the other fun stops along the body that is your pleasure trip, plus some tips on what to do when you hit one of these spots.

HIS EYES

We all know that men are visual creatures. Hello, just look at the multibillion-dollar porn industry, which lives and thrives because of it. Makes sense, doesn't it? The brain is the most powerful sexual organ (can't enjoy sex without it), and the eyes are directly wired into this all-important erogenous zone. So if you play to his sense of sight, you'll greatly enhance the sexual experience. Try having sex with the lights on, on top of the covers, and with your eyes open! Don't be afraid to look him in the eyes while doing all types of naughty things to him. Other fun ways to visually stimulate him include simply wearing sexy lingerie, doing a sensual dance for him, or masturbating while he watches.

TIPS FOR GIVING HIM A SEXY STRIPTEASE!

You don't have to know how to dance to do a striptease. Just use these key tips and give him a sight that he'll cherish forever:

- Select a song that moves you. Some ideas are "Hot in Herre" by Nelly for a hip-hop beat, "You Can Leave Your Hat On" by Joe Cocker for a seductive treat, or "Teach Me Tonight" by Dinah Washington for some old-time sensual charm. Whatever you do, don't lip synch the words; it looks silly!
- Dim the lights or set up candles or white holiday lights. Everything looks and feels better with the lights down low.
- Choose an outfit that looks and feels sexy. Wear five items—for example: a robe, booty shorts, a thong, and a bra. Don't forget to wear high heels!
- Make sure the outfit is easy to remove. You don't want to get bogged down by complicated straps or hooks.
- With the song as your accompaniment, slowly remove your clothing. Your movement doesn't have to be choreographed or complicated. Just move slowly and sway your hips.
- Take these words of famous 1930s striptease artist Gypsy Rose Lee to heart: "If it's worth doing, it's worth doing slowly . . . very slowly." This is the primary difference between a striptease and just taking your clothes off.
- Practice! Before showing off for your partner, do it in front of the mirror a few times so you can feel more confident when it comes to the real event.

- It's okay if you laugh (or even if he does!). You're only doing so because you're nervous. Just keep stripping, and the laughing will give way to something erotic.
- Tell him that you have a sexy surprise planned for him at 7 p.m. on Friday night and that he should be prepared. This way, he'll be in a very receptive mood. Don't try to surprise him with a striptease during his favorite sporting event or right after work.

HIS EARS

The pleasures you can bestow on your lover via the ear are manyfold. Try starting your foreplay with a little ear massage. Rubbing right behind the ear is an intimate and relaxing gesture and can provide just the right balance of sensations to get him in the mood. The skin on the outer ear is very sensitive; a soft blow, a tender kiss, or even a little nibble can be incredibly stimulating. Run your fingertips along the outermost edge of his ear, and then gently rub the lobe between your forefinger and thumb and tug on it a little. As you move inward, with a light touch or silken tongue, follow the concentric ridges and take your time. The physical sensation coupled with the sound will arouse him on different levels, which he may find incredibly erotic. The ear is *very* sensitive, so go slowly and ask him, in a sultry whisper, what he likes. Be careful, though: Nothing can gross a guy out and ruin the mood like a misplaced slurp right in the ear canal.

You can also stimulate him via the ears without ever touching him. We're referring to his sense of hearing, of course. For some men, nothing is more arousing than hearing a woman sigh and moan. "I was with a girl the other night, and she was going down on me. It wasn't very pleasurable at first, until I heard my roommate having sex in the next room. I could hear his partner moaning and crying out—the sound of her in there made me come almost immediately," says Dave, a 21-year-old student. The lesson here: Don't be afraid to get vocal. You don't have to be a screamer if you don't want to be, but don't hold back those sultry *mmm*s, *ohh*s, and *ahh*s.

And ladies, sometimes the sexiest thing you can do is utter a well-timed naughty statement. When said in an innocuous place, such as the frozen foods aisle of the grocery store, a sexy statement can create anticipation and serve as very effective foreplay. When said in the bedroom, it can be as pleasurable for him as a tweak of his nipple or a lick of his penis—especially if you don't already do it. We encourage you to cultivate your very own dirty-talk script.

Don't be surprised if by indulging in the art of dirty talk, you open up your vocabulary to include words that may have repulsed you before. Tara, a 33-year-old teacher, explains, "I used to absolutely hate the word *pussy*. To me, it was vulgar and insulting. So when a new lover said to me, 'I love the taste of your pussy,' I was not only surprised—I was shocked! But as our relationship progressed, his dirty words became an incredible turn-on to me, and I realized that some words hold amazing power as sexy, loving, and intimate."

SCRIPTING YOUR OWN DIRTY MONOLOGUE

Here are some deliciously naughty statements ranging from spicy to on fire! *Special note:* For some reason, for many men, adding the word *fuck* or *fucking* to your already naughty declarations has the same effect as when chef Emeril Lagasse adds his signature *Bam!* of spices to whatever he's cooking: It kicks it up a notch! Feel free to sprinkle your *Bam!* of *fucks* into your smutty statements as liberally or conservatively as you like. We've added stars in the following list where we think you could slip in some of this *fuck*-spice:

- Kiss me, you * sexy beast.
- I love the way your * cock tastes.
- Your * tongue feels so good on my * pussy.
- Fuck me.
- Ram my * pussy with your giant, hard cock.
- You are such a bad boy! I love it when you * touch me like that.

To make the dirty talk go smoothly, practice saying those naughty gems to yourself before unleashing them in the bedroom. This will cut down on the giggles or muffling of key syllables. Say them in the mirror to see how your mouth looks, and try different tones so you can pick the right sultry pitch. You'll find that the more you do it, the more easily the words will roll off of your tongue and the more colorful you'll get.

HIS NOSE

There's something to be said about the Eskimo kiss. It's not just a cutesy thing that the obnoxious couple does after the "I wub you" baby talk is exchanged. Interestingly, the nose contains a large amount of nerve endings, second only to the lips when it comes to the spots on his face. So gently rubbing noses can, in fact, be a sensual, stimulating act.

The nasal passages contain erectile tissue that expands with arousal (like another sexual body part we're pretty fond of), which actually causes nasal congestion. (The same is true for your own cute little button of a nose, but don't worry, this occurs mostly in the interior of the nasal passages.) It is thought that this reaction enhances the detection of pheromones. When the nose is mildly congested, inhalation produces little circular air currents within the nose, which causes more of whatever you are smelling to reach the olfactory epithelium (the scent sensors).[27] Slight congestion for him means that he'll smell more of your perfect pheromone cocktail, which in turn will increase his arousal.

We're not saying that a perfectly executed "nose job" will make him climax, but a nicely timed caress of his schnoz during kissing and foreplay will certainly serve to heighten his overall sexual experience.

HIS NIPPLES

Just because your nipples sit atop those luscious mammary glands of fatty tissue that are the object of every man's desire doesn't mean they are superior to men's when it comes to serving as vessels for pleasure-delivering nerve endings.

That's right, girls. Men's nipples, and the surrounding tissue, are every bit as sensitive as yours, which makes them fabulous body parts to tickle, pinch, kiss, lick, and bite. A study published in *The Journal of Sexual Medicine* in May 2006 reported that for 51.7 percent of men, "nipple stimulation caused or enhanced their sexual arousal."[28]

The important lesson to take away is that men's responses, just like women's, will be varied, but for the most part positive. For some men, nipple stimulation is pleasant. For some, it is hot. And for others, it is the ultimate trigger to take them over the climactic threshold. Likewise, some like it when you lick, some prefer a nice pinch, and some want a touch of teeth. As in all things, experiment and ask!

FUN TOOLS TO USE IN OFF-THE-COCK EXPLORATIONS

While navigating his erogenous map, try using more than just your hands and mouth. Give these tips a shot:

- Break out the scented massage oil and give your man a full-body massage, from his neck to the soles of his feet. Linger on every square inch of skin and discover the hiding places of *all* his secret spots.

- Use a feather to lightly caress his skin. Try tickling the nape of his neck, his sides, and the small of his back— all these areas are packed with nerve endings. Linger in a spot when he gives you encouragement, but move on if he starts to squirm uncomfortably.

- Use body massage candles to add a warm sensation to your sex play. Drip the wax from these specially designed candles onto his skin and then massage it in. We don't recommend using traditional wax candles for this, because they will burn!

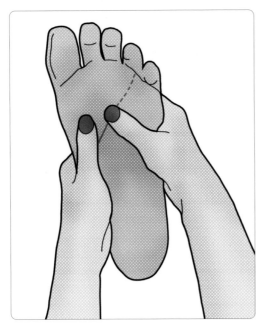

THE SOLE OF HIS FOOT ◄

When it comes to tripping alternative triggers on his body, the bottom of his foot is another sweet spot. Chinese medicine tells us that the "Bubbling Spring" acupressure point can be found just below the ball of the foot, within the sole. Some believe that pressing this point creates "bubbling" sensations that rise up through his legs and into his genitals. But more important, the sole of the foot, like every other erotic trigger on the body, contains a large concentration of nerve endings and is thus sensitive to massage as well as tickling.

 TIP:

Use a little bit of warming lube in your hands and massage it in circular motions on the sole of his foot, pausing every so often to press just below the ball of his foot in the center. Warming and caressing this sweet spot will both relax and titillate him, and if there's any truth to the "Bubbling Spring" point, you'll have that covered as well.

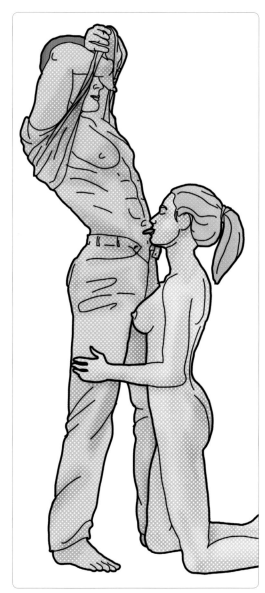

Lick and kiss down his "Sea of Energy."

HIS BELLY BUTTON ◄

Let us begin with a warning: Tread lightly here! There appears to be a mysterious connection between the belly button and the penis, at least for some men. Scientific data that provides a reason for this phenomenon is hard to come by, but word on our personal investigative street is that it exists. For most men, the connection is not a pleasant one.[29] The majority of the men we interviewed who had any reaction to navel physical stimulation said it was unpleasant— that pressing the belly button created an almost painful sensation in the tip of the penis. Others said touching the belly button did nothing for them. And very, very few said that pressing on the belly button during arousal and climax actually accentuated the experience. Because the information is spotty, we recommend that you deliberately ask your lover how it feels as you caress or press on his navel—if he hasn't already slapped your hand away!

However, 2 to 3 inches (5.08 to 7.62 cm) below the navel is a row of reflexology points known as the "Sea of Energy," which is linked to his erotic engine and fertility.[30] Trail a string of sensual kisses from his belly button down to his forest of fun and see if you can get his Sea of Energy roiling into a nice storm.

Chapter **7**

TOYS FOR BOYS

WHY USE SEX TOYS WHEN HE ALREADY HAS A DIRTY T-SHIRT AND VASELINE?

Let's be honest: Most men don't go beyond a lubed up palm and a sock during their solo sex-plorations. Says Jim, a 20-something programmer, "If I'm paying a hundred dollars for a toy, I may as well double down and get a prostitute."

However, there seems to be a respectable number of men out there who are open and willing to include sex toys in their lives. In our sex survey, 36 percent of men reported that they use sex toys designed for men while masturbating, and 34 percent said they use them during partner play.

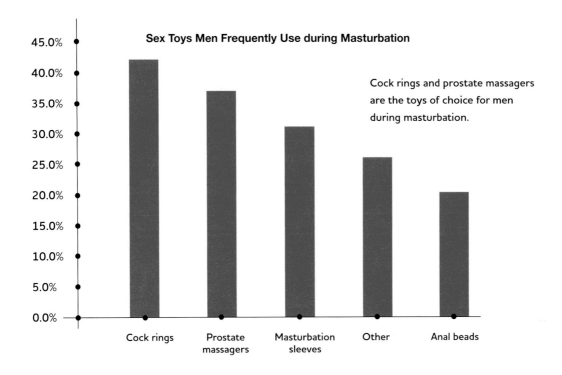

Sex Toys Men Frequently Use during Masturbation

Cock rings and prostate massagers are the toys of choice for men during masturbation.

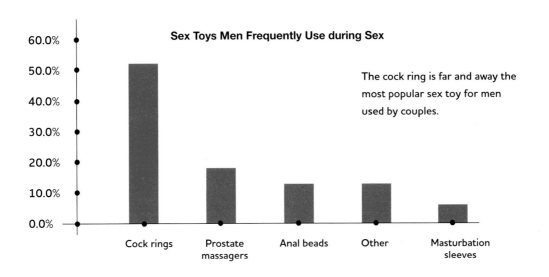

Sex Toys Men Frequently Use during Sex

The cock ring is far and away the most popular sex toy for men used by couples.

If your guy is one of the 64 percent of men who don't touch the things, it may be time to stock up on AA batteries and turn him on to a whole new world of pleasure. With an ever-growing selection of toys designed for him on the market, starting a collection is easy, and it's a great way to add variety to your bedroom games. As cited by Dr. Dick, some benefits of sex toys are that they'll increase his sexual repertoire, improve his all-over body awareness, and facilitate prostate massage.

In this chapter, we will investigate what types of sex toys are out there for him, what they do for him, what they do for you, and how to use them.

LUBRICANT (BECAUSE WET SEX IS BETTER THAN DRY HUMPING)

Lube is the single most important sex toy out there—and for a typical guy, it's the *only* sex toy he'll ever use when masturbating! Says Troy, a 34-year-old designer, "Over time, I've experimented with a lot of lubes. My favorite choice is cheap lotion paired with a dirty T-shirt: inexpensive enough to masturbate daily with, and it works."

Dr. Dick says:

"Sometimes it's difficult getting straight men to warm up to the idea of incorporating toys for themselves in partnered play. They can also be resistant to toys for solo play. Some think toys are gay or only for women. Some haven't a large enough sexual repertoire to even imagine how toys could assist them or be fun."

While cheap lotion may work for masturbation sessions, it probably won't work well for partner play. And without proper lube, there's not much you can do with any of the toys listed in this chapter. So which lube is right for which sticky sexual situation?

SILICONE-BASED LUBE

Silicone-based lube is an excellent option for hand jobs and anal play because it is longer lasting and won't get sticky like water-based lube. It's also great to use if you're looking for a little playtime in the shower or bath because it won't rinse away with water; you'll need to scrub with soap and water to wash it off. Also, silicone-based lube won't harm toys or condoms. However, if you plan to use this type of lube during vaginal intercourse, make sure you invest in a brand that's paraben- and glycerin-free. Those two ingredients can mess with the pH levels of your vagina, resulting in a yeast infection. Ew. Our favorite silicone lube? Wet Naturals Silky Supreme.

WATER-BASED LUBES

If your hand jobs or toy play often result in intercourse and you don't want to worry about your delicate pH balance, we recommend a water-based lube. Water-based lubes are compatible with toys and condoms, and rinse away with water. When it gets sticky, just reapply. Our favorite water-based lube? Astroglide.

OIL- AND PETROLEUM-BASED LUBES

Oil- and petroleum-based lubricants include things you can find around the house, such as the time-tested Jergens lotion. We don't recommend using these, especially if you plan on having sex after all of that handsy fun. Oil- and petroleum-based lubes degrade condoms and diaphragms and can irritate the vagina.

SOAP

Nothing is simpler or slipperier than a spontaneous game of manual manipulation in the bath or shower with plenty of body soap. However, be sure to wash the soap off completely if you move on to intercourse, and don't use shampoo because it can irritate your honey's sensitive urethra.

NATURAL SECRETIONS—YOURS OR HIS!

Some men generate a lot of pre-cum when sexually stimulated. If your guy is one of these, use his secretions as lubrication. Alternatively, or in addition, you can use your saliva or even your vaginal secretions to create a slippery situation. Your saliva or his pre-cum is a particularly good choice if you ever spontaneously lend him a hand, say, during the halftime show for the Super Bowl.

LUBE ON THE GO

For those of you who happen upon random sex play at regular intervals, you may opt to carry sample-size packets of lube in your purse. We don't recommend carrying bottles around; if you do, you may have to explain the sticky wad of singles you pull out of your purse when you pay the dry cleaner.

DOUBLE-DUTY LUBES

Want to make that blow job more pleasurable for you? Use a flavored lube! There are all kinds of water-soluble, edible lubes in an array of interesting flavors. We'll be honest, girls, not all of these "flavors" are accurate, but at the end of the day, they can taste a whole lot better than eight-hour-old penis sweat.

Want to make that blow job even more pleasurable for him? Try an edible cooling lube. Put a dab on your tongue and go to town. The cooling lube will create the sensation that you have ice cubes in your mouth. Edible lubes also come with warming properties (these provide the *sensation* of warmth—they won't burn your tongue) and fizzing properties (think: giving head with a mouthful of Pop Rocks candy). Some lubes have stimulating properties when rubbed on the head of the penis (note that these usually also feel awesome on the clitoris), and others claim to have aphrodisiacal ingredients, which supposedly make you even hornier when licking his stick. We recommend going the hippy route when it comes to edible lubes: Look for organic, all-natural, paraben-free, petrochemical-free (you get the picture) products.

Of course, all sorts of magical lube properties can be found in nonedible lubes, too. The sky is the limit on how you might use them. Just be sure to use common sense and follow the guidelines we've established for what types of lubes should be used with what sex acts.

TOYS YOU CAN PUT ON HIS PECKER

The penis is often the mission control center for the male sex experience, so it makes sense to give his rod some fun with titillating sex toys. Here are some exciting devices that you can put on his pecker.

COCK RINGS ▼

The cock ring is the most popular toy used by our survey-takers: 54 percent of male sex-toy users in our survey have worn one during intercourse, and 43 percent have worn one during masturbation. This little device is worn around the base of his erect penis and hugs the shaft tightly, preventing blood from easily escaping the erection. To put it on, just lube him up and slide it on. The result? A harder hard-on that lasts longer.

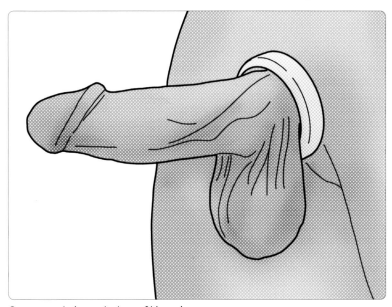

Secure a cock ring at the base of his penis.

In addition to a raging hard-on, cock rings offer a variety of sensual enhancements for both partners. They come in metal, latex, rubber, leather, and silicon. There are nubbed ones and studded ones and black, red, and glow-in-the-dark ones. Some even have clit rubbers, vibrators, prostrate massagers, buckles, leashes, or lassos. With so many options, you'll find that you and your partner have a lot of experimenting to do. With the added bonus of most rings being priced at under ten dollars, you could have several inexpensive date nights to remember!

MASTURBATION SLEEVES ▼

If he's not jealous of your jelly dildo, you shouldn't envy his masturbation sleeve! These squishy tubes are intended to replicate the sensation of sliding his erection into a warm, slippery place . . . such as a vagina. In our survey, 31 percent of male sex-toy users told us they use sleeves to enhance their masturbation sessions, but only 6 percent said they use them during partner play. That's too bad, because they make hand jobs easy work for you. Some girls also reported that they've cheated

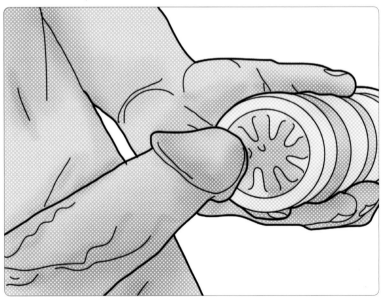

Slide a masturbation sleeve over his erect penis.

on blow jobs by slipping one of these lubed up devices over his cock and letting it do the "hard work" for them. With the lights out, he may never be the wiser! Mutual masturbation is also greatly enhanced using these fun little suckers.

Sleeves come in a variety of shapes, sizes, textures, and materials. Some are meant to be handheld and used for masturbation or assisted masturbation. Others actually slip over the shaft of the penis and are thin enough to allow room for cock-into-pussy action. This type of sleeve is often equipped with nubs or ribs that enhance your sensation during intercourse. Other types of sleeves are reversible and can be used both ways.

THE ORO STIMULATOR ▼

This male sex toy was brought to our attention as a resident in the catchall "other" category of sex toys. Basically a suction cup with a pump, the Oro Stimulator attempts to recreate the sensation of a blow job. This is one brand in a long line of these types of toys, some of which are molded after a woman's lips. Is this a cry for more blow jobs, or what?

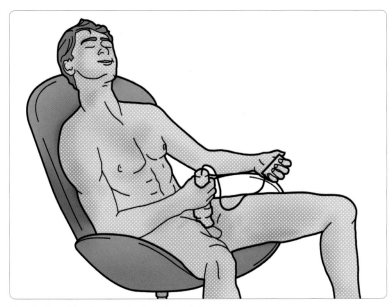

Use the Oro Stimulator to simulate a blow job.

TOYS YOU CAN PUT IN HIS BUTT

Let's move beyond the penis, shall we? If you've read chapter 5, "Funky Butt Lovin' and the P-Spot," you're well aware that your man's ass is a treasure trove of pleasure. Here we discuss toys that will help you penetrate his secret cavern.

ANAL BEADS ▼

The classic version of these surprisingly delectable devices features plastic beads laced on a string, with a finger-sized loop handle at the end. Newer versions look like an octopus tentacle with beads held together in a bendable column of jelly material. Some strands feature beads that incrementally increase in size.

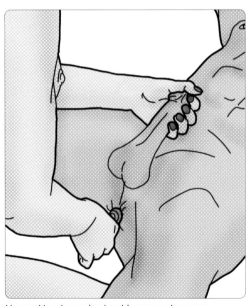 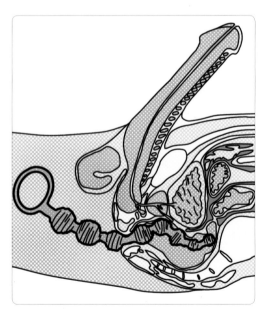

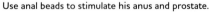
Use anal beads to stimulate his anus and prostate.

As the name suggests, the idea is to poke the beads up his bum. While you are manipulating his cock with your hand or mouth, lube up his butthole and insert one bead at a time. If he can handle it, don't stop until you've inserted the whole strand! As your guy comes, slowly pull the beads out and watch him experience an unbelievably heightened orgasm.

BUTT PLUGS ▼

These miniature, volcano-shaped cones work a lot better than a lightbulb in the butt. They used to come in three sizes (small, medium, and large) and two colors (flesh and black), but now they come in such a wide array of shapes, sizes, colors, and materials that it can be dizzying to decide just which of these doodads would best fit in your honey's holy hole. We suggest you start small and cheap, and if he's into it, slowly graduate to larger or more sophisticated versions (for example, the more

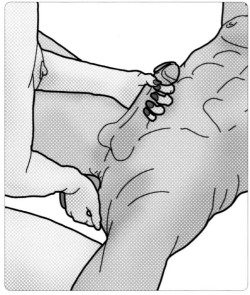 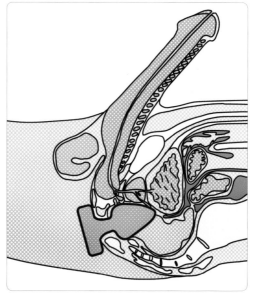

Make sure the butt plug you use for anal play has a flared bottom.

expensive glass plugs are delightful because they can be warmed up or cooled for added sensation). Make certain that whatever you choose has a wide base so you can secure the plug in place and ensure that it won't disappear up his hoo-ha. Just lube it up, slip it in, and then ride his cock or pay attention to other parts of his body. The pressure against his prostate will add tremendous zing to his ejaculation.

PROSTATE MASSAGERS ▼

The aliens have landed and are taking over his uncharted territory. Prostate massagers are sci fi–looking devices that swoop and swirl and aim to effectively stimulate this oft-ignored erogenous zone.

In our sex survey, 39 percent of men who use toys during masturbation enjoy toys that massage their prostates, and just a lonely 18 percent said they've used these devices when partnered with a pretty lady. This is unfortunate, because a prostate massager is an excellent option for the girl who's squeamish about putting her dainty digit in his not-so-dainty derriere.

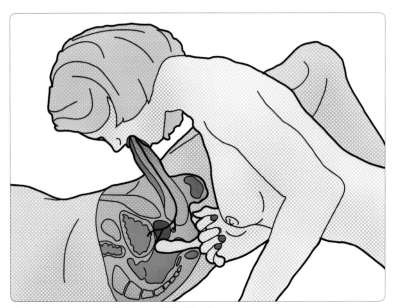

Use a prostate massager in tandem with a blow job.

Poke one of these lubed-up devices in his butt and massage his prostate and perineum with it while you perform oral sex. Literally, you'll have him wrapped around a toy, but figuratively, he'll be wrapped around your finger. (Seriously. What do you want? A diamond? A sports car? Now's the time to ask.) A vibrating stimulator adds a whole lot of screaming pleasure and can rev his engine into overdrive.

There are quite a few prostate massagers designed by doctors on the market, which is another indicator of just how important prostate massage is for prostate health. Many of these are designed to give a massage of the same medical quality as one given by a urologist, without the hospital gown and rubber glove (unless you two are into that scene), with the added bonus of providing him with an incredible orgasm.

For the anal play novice, many of these toys can look a bit intimidating. Men who are not used to being penetrated in the derriere may think that several of the models out there look absolutely huge, which is something we ladies may overlook since we're accustomed to penetration by much larger objects. Not to worry. Dr. Emmey tells us that if your guy doesn't have to go it alone, a finger in the butt is a perfectly pleasurable way to deliver that healthful prostate massage. No toys necessary. Read chapter 5, "Funky Butt Lovin' and the P-Spot," for more information on proper technique.

STRAP-ONS AND DILDOS

We consider the strap-on to be the big daddy of all sex toys for him. Why is this? Well, for one, it turns the tables and enables you to be the big daddy in the bedroom. For another, it's one of those toys that is considered pretty wild and taboo, even for men who enjoy anal stimulation. Case in point: David, a 30-year-old stockbroker who loves anal stimulation and frequently gives his lovers guidance on how to properly massage his prostate, vehemently declares, "I will absolutely never let a woman fuck me in the ass with a strap-on!"

The man who enjoys being pegged by his female lover is a rare (and we think wonderful) bird, indeed. Whether your sweetie is only curious or already a full-fledged devotee, there are some important things to keep in mind.

A strap-on is a device that you wear on your crotch (think something like a chastity belt, but you hold the key) that enables you to make love to your man as if you were . . . well . . . a man.

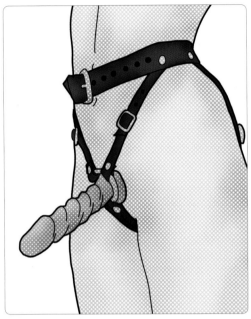

Use a strap-on to peg your man.

The strap-on holds the dildo of your choosing in place, so be sure pick a strap-on that is comfortable enough to wear as long as you both want to go. You don't want to have to stop the fun because of a little chafing!

Strap-ons come in a variety of styles. Some look like panties, some look rather "strappy," and some even have vibrating clitoral stimulation as well! You can purchase all-in-one, packaged strap-ons with fake cock included, but if you're going for quality, we recommend buying the strap-on and dildo separately. In addition, if you're planning on taking your man anally more than once or twice, you should invest in a quality product made of leather, imitation leather, or high-grade vinyl. There are also strap-ons that attach to the thigh, which allow for more interesting and creative positioning.

Choose a dildo that is a good fit for your lover. Be thoughtful, ladies. If he's new to this whole thing, don't get a ten-inch cock monster! And just as we hope he treats you with penile penetration, we hope you don't give him the ol' wham, bam, thank you, *man*! Take your time, make sure he's fully aroused and enjoying himself, use plenty of lube, maybe warm him up with a finger or a smaller butt plug, and when you're finally ready to give a good thrusting, go slow. That is, until you hear those telltale words: "Harder! Faster!"

TOYS OF A DIFFERENT FEATHER

In our sex survey, 14 percent of men described using other types of sex toys during sex, and 26 percent used something else during masturbation. So what's in this "other" category? Some of these "other" items include the more commonplace dildos and vibrators. Interestingly, many of these toys are tools used in the BDSM lifestyle (which could take up a whole book in and of itself).

BLINDFOLDS, WAX, RESTRAINTS, AND NIPPLE CLAMPS

Ah, the lighter side of bondage and domination! These toys are often used by people who are into BDSM, but they're also wonderfully fun as what we like to call "tourist attractions" (see chapter 11, "The Kinkster"). Each of these, when used in a playful way, can heighten his sexual experience. Taking away his sight with a blindfold enhances his other senses so that every touch and every sound you make can become a sensual surprise. Tie his hands and watch him squirm as you lick, kiss, bite, and caress according to your every whim—and he has the pleasure of being taken for a ride. Hot wax employs just enough danger and spice to make the session oh so naughty. And ladies, nipple clamps can be used simply to stimulate and put pressure on his nipples while you tend to other areas. They don't have to inflict pain (unless he wants it).

THE PARACHUTE

This medieval-looking device is made of leather decorated in metal studs and is shaped somewhat like its namesake. It is billed as a "cock-and-ball torture device." Slip your man's testicles into the opening and tighten that bad-boy parachute up as much as you are able to. The device comes with chains meant to hold weights up to three pounds! This toy is one of the many varieties of full-blown bondage gear used in BDSM, and it is really meant to be used with your submissive kinkster, should you have one. Good luck trying to get your vanilla or dominant lover to squeeze his grapes into one of these things!

ELECTRO-STIMULATION PRODUCTS

Does your guy get a charge out of testicular electrocution? If so, he's into erotic electro-stimulation. With their generators, wires, and frequency switches, these devices look like something you'd find in Dr. Frankenstein's laboratory. The idea is to deliver low-frequency shocks to the body, usually focused on the genitals. The focusing devices (i.e., the parts that actually touch the body) come in all toy forms, from cock rings to anal plugs to devices that simulate deep throating, but they all deliver a spark that will have you crying out "It's *ALIVE*!" The recommended lube for these products? Olive oil.

Chapter 8

HIS LIBIDO: UNDERSTANDING YOUR HORNBALL

IN THE WORLD OF MALE SEXUALITY, there are many forces that can affect his sexual desire and performance. Genetics, his diet, his workout regime, cultural expectations, pheromones, hormones, and Viagra are just some of the forces that your guy may encounter. Men aren't as sexually simple as we think, and it's best to arm yourself with the knowledge of what makes his sex life tick. May the force be with you!

THE MALE SEX DRIVE—*VROOM, VROOM!*

Picture the male sex drive like a car, the one he got for his sixteenth birthday. He may be the flashy owner of a sleek, speedy sports car, or he may be the quieter owner of an economical hybrid. He may have an endless supply of gas money, or he may have to painstakingly save up his pennies for every mile he drives. His car may attract bevies of girls who enjoy cruising down Main Street, or he may choose one lady to take on a long, adventurous road trip. The thing about this car is, whether he likes it or not, he's got it for life. And depending on how well he takes care of it, and whether he gets in any accidents, the car will either run for life or it will end up in a junk heap.

If his sex drive were indeed a car, testosterone would be the gasoline that fuels it. Men produce anywhere from ten to forty times more testosterone than women. Its function is to generate sperm and regulate sex drive. It also causes five o'clock shadows, big muscles, and hairy toes. Throughout a man's life, his sex drive will remain pretty stable, as long as he is in good health. So if he starts out with an active sex drive overflowing with testosterone, he'll likely remain that way throughout his life. Sure, his testosterone levels and baseline sex drive will decrease with age, but the decrease will be

Dr. Glenda says:

"Women think male sexuality is simple. The analogy that always gets touted around is 'Men are like bicycles and women are like jet airplanes.' Male sexuality is assumed to operate on a very simple hydraulic principle. Get it up, get it in, get it off, get it up again! It's pretty much assumed that for women, if they show up and he doesn't get off, something is amiss. Women often don't understand that it may require more than a couple of strokes and a little spit."

gradual and may not even be noticeable. However, if he is the guy who started out driving the less-powerful hybrid and his sex drive diminishes from mild to poor, the change may be more obvious.

Do you want to find out whether your guy has a lot of testosterone? Scientists suggest you check his ring finger. The longer it is in relation to his index finger, the more testosterone he has. According to the SEX I.D. test conducted by a team of psychologists for the BBC, a typical index-to-ring-finger ratio for men is about 0.96, and women are closer to 1.00 (meaning the two fingers are about the same length).[31]

SEX DRIVE VERSUS SEX FUNCTION

If sex drive is the vehicle, then sex function is the road he travels. A man who has a fully operational race car–type sex drive to begin with can still get stuck in the rut of poor sex function. But if he makes the right turns, he could speed freely down horny highway. Unlike the drive (or libido), which is the man's innate desire for sex and is internally regulated by hormones, sex function is his physical and psychological ability to perform. This is vulnerable to an assortment of outside influences.

In the O&C sex survey, men cited that regular exercise greatly improved their desire for sex and their ability to function. Says Jim, a 45-year-old architect, "I'm a runner, and when I'm training consistently, my drive follows my weekly mileage—up, up, up."

On the flip side, alcohol was the culprit behind most men's inability to perform. Says 64-year-old George, "Alcohol makes me think I'm amorous but renders me ineffectual."

The lesson here? If you want your guy to be in tip-top sexual function, ask him to lay off the booze and pick up the running shoes!

YOUR GUY IS ON A SOLAR CYCLE

Pagans were on to something when they called the moon a goddess and the sun a god. As it turns out, just as women go through a monthly hormonal cycle that corresponds to the tides of the moon, men go through a daily cycle that is similar to the rising and setting of the sun. A study conducted by S.J. Winters et al. at the University of Pittsburgh determined that men's testosterone levels are highest in the morning and lowest in the evening, higher in the fall and lower in the spring.[32] So anytime your guy starts acting like a grumpy pants, you can reach over, pat him on the back, and ask, "Oh honey, is it that time of the day again?"

LET'S FACE IT: MEN WANT MORE SEX (OR AT LEAST THEY THINK THEY DO!)

Our men admit it: They constantly think about "hitting it," "screwing it," and "nailing it," even when they're not working construction. A significant 92 percent of the men we surveyed said they think about sex several times per day or more! And most men wish they were having more sex then they currently are. It seems that a guy who is getting laid once per week wishes he were going at it two to three times per week, and the guy who's lucky enough to get a daily dose wishes for it multiple times per day. We call this reality/desire formula the "randy rule," which says, the more sex you get, the more sex you want.

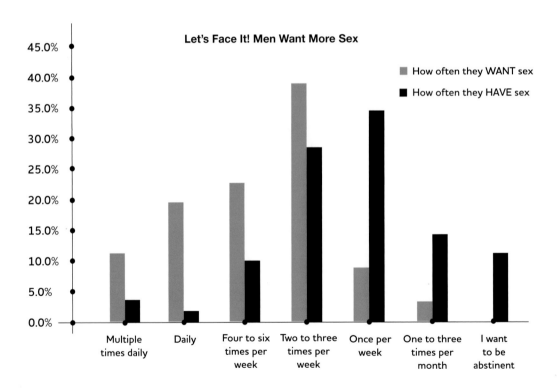

So do men want more sex than women do? In the O&C sex survey, 64 percent of men said they want sex more often than their partners do. Of the ladies surveyed, only 27 percent said their man wants more sex than they do. Where does this disparity come from? Why do men say that they want more sex than women, but women disagree? (It certainly could be because our informal survey was created and compiled by nonscientists—no lab rats, white coats, or beakers were used or harmed in the making of this survey!).

One possible theory is that there is often a huge communication disconnect between men and women. There are likely millions of couples around the world who aren't leading a fulfilling sex life simply because they don't realize that their partner wants sex, too!

Another plausible reason is that, in our culture, men learn that they are supposed to be up for sex anytime, anywhere, with little more stimulation than a glimpse of cleavage. When they don't live up to this unrealistic "norm," they don't want to admit it. Dr. Glenda tells us that the unintended consequence of the belief in the invincible male sex drive is that it has become a social reality, whether it's true or not. Like the Thomas theorem states: If something is defined as real, it is real in its consequences. Consequently, men believe that to be a true man, as defined by our culture, they must also be incorrigible horndogs, incapable of keeping their minds out of the gutter and their penises in their pants.

Dr. Jenni says:

"A lot of women think that men are the ones with the higher sex drive and that they always want sex. But in reality, there are plenty of times when men will say, 'Eh, not tonight, honey.' The myth of the unstoppable male sex drive may be one of our culture's biggest misconceptions."

SURPRISE! YOUR GUY HAS FEELINGS

Although his penis may demand a lot of attention during sex, it's actually your guy's brain that is the most important sex organ. You may be surprised to hear that 72 percent of men we surveyed said they prefer to have an emotional connection during sex. Says 50-something Joe, "No emotional connection, no erection."

For women who are insecure about their men going to strip clubs, take heart in what Samuel, a 40-something executive, says: "I can be intimate with my wife and can 'get it up' when needed. Funny, because in a 'gentlemen's club' a sexy woman may be grinding on my crotch, but nothing . . ."

Many other men told us that they'd prefer to have sex with a doll or just do it themselves rather than have sex for the sake of fucking.

It's critical to understand that emotions and romantic ideals are very often an important part of a man's sexual experience. Without tapping in to his head and heart, women can't even begin to understand a man's sexual potential.

Dr. Jenni says:

"Sometimes we overlook a man's mental and emotional sex drive. Believe it or not, sometimes men don't want sex because they may be mentally or emotionally disconnected from their partner . . . Let's not forget that men have a sex drive between their ears, too."

THE SECRETS OF ATTRACTION

What is it about women that attracts men most? Is it their eyes? Smile? Personality? Bangin' bod? Out of more than two hundred men who answered this question, 32 percent said it is her personality, while 29 percent told us it is her physical assets. Says 40-something Robert, "Initially, obviously, it's the appearance. That's a threshold issue. After that, she must be intelligent and have an appealing personality. Noticeably lacking any of the three qualities kills the attraction."

Most men went on to explain that they really prefer "the whole package" and that sometimes their attraction to a woman is completely intangible, that it's just "something about her."

There are so many articles out there about whether men prefer skinny chicks or bootylicious babes, whether they prefer blondes or brunettes, tall girls or short. We just want to set the record straight: Every man is an individual with his own desires and attractions, and of course there is always a level of fluidity in what he wants. A gentleman who prefers blondes may also find his heart aflutter when he meets that sassy brunette next door. The nature of attraction is so mysterious that it's a waste of time to try to fit any mold. The most important steps you can take are to stay healthy, be confident, and make good choices about the men you invite into your boudoir!

THE SCENT OF SEX: DO PHEROMONES EXIST?

If you ask a scientist about the nature of attraction, she may tell you that it's all about chemical and hormonal reactions, that physical and mental desire is really just an illusion. Pheromones are possible key players in this reaction.

Dr. Hiroaki Matsunami of Duke University defines pheromones as "chemicals that can affect innate behaviors or hormonal levels." According to Dr. Matsunami's research, the human pheromone is a sex steroid compound called androstenone, and it can be found in sweat, saliva, and urine. He postulates that humans can actually smell these chemicals, and depending on your genetic makeup (and, we assume, that of the person whose armpit you are sniffing), the odor will either be appealing, revolting, or neutral.[33]

The lesson? We should all act more like dogs in our approach to mingling with the opposite sex. Before wasting money on that first cocktail, much less a brand-new outfit or an expensive dinner, each of you should lift your arms and take a big whiff of the other (be sure not to wear deodorant!). If the two of you like what you smell, go home and mate. Wouldn't that make the whole dating game a lot easier?

Turns out it's not that simple. Even the science types aren't 100 percent sure what role these chemicals play in our love lives. In an attempt to determine the power of pheromones, researchers from the University of Bern in Switzerland asked a group of women to smell unwashed T-shirts that had been worn by six different men for two full nights. The women unknowingly sniffed out and rejected shirts whose owners they were closely related to, saying that the odor was smelly and offensive. The women were most attracted to the tees of the guys who had very different immune systems from their own, a genetic condition which would allow for the healthiest offspring. They also often noted that those "good-smelling" T-shirts reminded them of their past lovers.

Women who were on birth control pills experienced the opposite effect, preferring the scent of men whose genetics were more similar to their own. Researchers postulate that, because the pill tricks the body into thinking it's already pregnant, women under that hormonal influence are seeking the shelter of "family members" (those to whom they are genetically related) for security during gestation. One could imagine far-reaching consequences of this study; for example, if you started the pill during the middle of your relationship, would your partner, who once smelled like delicious sex on a stick, suddenly have the aroma of stinky French cheese?[34]

This 1995 study showed that women are sensitive to his pheromonal odor. But what about men? In 2002, researchers at the University of Mexico repeated this study but included men in the research. They found that men strongly preferred the scent of women who were at fertile points in their cycles, and that they also preferred women who had dissimilar immunity genes.[35] So it seems there is something to be said about the scent of a woman, after all!

With science beginning to back evidence of the importance of pheromones and DNA in attraction, entrepreneurs have sought to capitalize on it. For example, the dating site ScientificMatch .com charges $1,995.95 for a lifetime membership. Mail in cheek swabs for your DNA, and it will make matches with people based upon compatible personality values and DNA samples.

Other companies have bottled synthetic pheromones, claiming that they help you attract people of the opposite sex. The effectiveness of these synthetic pheromones has yet to be fully verified. However, in 2005, the ABC television show *20/20* did a piece in which identical twins attended a speed-dating event, one wearing pheromones, one not. They each went on ten five-minute dates. At the end of the night, the twin who wore the pheromones received nine follow-up date requests, and the one who didn't only received five.[36]

THE SEVEN-YEAR-ITCH

While pheromones help attract your guy to your sexy gene pool in the first place, there are other chemicals that are responsible for the success of your relationship. Both men and women experience the same sequence of events. For that first, hot rush of love, a chemical combination of dopamine, norepinephrine, and phenylethylamine floods your brain—a very addictive cocktail indeed. This high ultimately wears off as your brain becomes accustomed to the particular combination of chemicals, which leads to that experience often referred to as the seven-year itch (though it's a bit of a misnomer, as it actually takes six months to two years for the puppy-love cocktail to wear off). In the words of B.B. King, you may feel that "the thrill is gone." However, if your relationship survives and proceeds beyond this shift, you'll both experience an onset of new chemicals: oxytocin and vasopressin. These bring the warm fuzzy feeling of love, and generate an attachment that, if treated properly and given the opportunity (with plenty of romance and creative sex), can last forever.[37]

ERECTIONS IN A BOTTLE: VIAGRA, CIALIS, AND LEVITRA

Our culture is obsessed with erections. How else can you explain the Washington Monument? We love erections so much that we think of a man who can't get it up as being impotent (or powerless). But did you know that erections aren't always directly correlated to his arousal? In the O&C sex survey, 68 percent of the men said that within the past year they have experienced an erection *without* the desire for sex, and 74 percent of our men have been aroused without an erection! This hasn't stopped drug companies from making a mad dash to facilitate the more erect erection and capitalizing on our love for boners.

In the early 1990s, a group of scientists at Pfizer were testing a compound called sildenafil citrate, which was intended to help cardiovascular health by improving blood flow to the heart. The drug apparently didn't do much for the heart, but it caused an unintended side effect in its test subjects: damn good erections. When the boner-shaped opportunity knocked, drug companies answered. Realizing the potential demand for harder hard-ons, Pfizer created Viagra. In 1998, the FDA approved this miracle drug, and men began popping the little blue pills in a valiant effort to combat erectile dysfunction (ED), whether they had it or not. Dr. Jenni says that Viagra is one of the most overprescribed medications out there. "Many of the users don't suffer from true organic erectile dysfunction. Many get it from friends because they hear they can last longer," she says.

Organic ED is a strictly physical problem caused by conditions such as diabetes, high cholesterol, and obesity that inhibit blood flow to the penis. But Dr. Jenni tells us that most men who can't get it up are usually experiencing some form of performance anxiety. She explains, "I encourage my clients to learn natural skills to be able to last longer and not to depend on Viagra. A lot of men psychologically trick themselves to believe they need Viagra to have sex."

In 1999, the first major Viagra ad campaign featured a sober Bob Dole speaking out about the hardships of living with ED (a term which, by the way, was invented alongside Viagra). The marketing powers knew that few men would want to admit to what was heretofore known as impotence and would much prefer to blame their sex woes on a dysfunctional erection.[38]

Dr. Jenni says:

"To be clear, men can't just take a pill and go home, watch TV, and experience a pop-up erection . . . They still have to have some form of arousal for the medication to work."

In the following decade, other brands of ED meds hit the prescription pads, including Cialis and Levitra. Competing ads for all three drugs made their way to prime-time spots, mostly during sporting events, and often featured middle-aged gentlemen, with full heads of hair, smiling and laughing with their partners in anticipation of a sexy evening or in the afterglow of sex.

Recently, the men in these commercials are becoming younger and visually more virile male specimens. YouTube hosts an array of humorous ED medication videos that show men doing hands-free push-ups on their penises and steering cars with their erections. Comedian Robin Williams described ED drugs as drugs "to make you harder than Chinese Algebra!" The result? ED drugs have become mainstream, and more and younger users are trying them. In the O&C sex survey, 28 percent of the male participants told us they have taken ED medicine, and 18 percent of those admitted they took it just for fun. Several respondents told us they like to pop an ED pill if they're put in a particularly sexy situation, such as a threesome, where they may be expected to last longer.

Real-life users report varying degrees of the drug's effectiveness. Most of our respondents who have tried the drug were pleased with the results. Jerry, a 30-something admin, says, "I walked around with an erection for hours. She couldn't keep up with me! But I had a great time." A lot of men reported that Viagra is much more intense than Cialis, but that it sometimes gives them headaches and flushed faces. However, although the three drugs are made by three different companies and have different active ingredients, they generally perform the same function—specifically, to relax the smooth muscles in his penis, allowing more blood to pump into his pecker.

Is there danger in using the drugs recreationally? Yes, of course. As with all drugs, prescription and otherwise, there are often side effects. The FDA has reported several cases of sudden hearing loss from individuals who've used ED drugs. A serious potential side effect from the misuse of an ED drug is priapism, which is an erection that won't go away.[39] In season one, episode four of *True Blood*, Jason Stackhouse (Ryan Kwanten) overdoses on vampire blood and experiences an erection that just won't quit. He ends up in the emergency room, where a doctor takes a giant needle to his johnson and drains the excess blood. In extreme cases of priapism, this is exactly what the ER doctor will do. If untreated, priapism can cause the penis to scar and create long-term, organic ED. Ironic, isn't it?

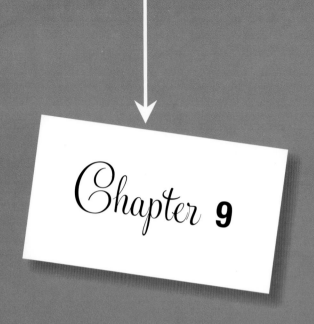

Chapter **9**

HIS BRAIN ON SEX: PORN, RELIGION, AND TABOOS

AS MUCH AS WE WISH IT WEREN'T SO, social standards, influences, and taboos inevitably make their wily way into the boudoir. In the grand scheme of possible negative influences that may affect your sex life, some seem like opposing forces. In one corner, weighing 325 pounds and made up of so many hours of digital downloads, scratched DVDs, and spent videotape, is every porno flick your lover has ever seen. And in the other corner, weighing close to two tons, is the elephant in the room that feasts on religious and social taboos. When these two opposing forces go at it, you've got the equivalent of the 1997 Holyfield-Tyson fight in the middle of your bedroom. Someone is bound to lose an ear.

WHAT'S UP WITH PORN?

Porn films firmly made their way into American consciousness in the 1970s. Dr. Glenda says, "The adult industry began as a social movement in the '70s. Adult filmmakers saw it as a liberation movement about bringing sexuality out into the open."

Out in the open it is, indeed. Unless you've been living in a nunnery your whole adult life, chances are you've watched a porn film at one time or another. You are likely familiar with the monstrously large appendages plunging into perfectly shaven porn-star pussies, the fake boobs, the cheesy music, the four-hour fuckfests, the money shots—in short, the grandiose *performance* of it all. And you may or may not have a problem with it.

Ladies, love it or hate it, pornography is here to stay, especially when it comes to your man. It behooves you to address whatever personal problems you may have with porn, be they feminist, postmodernist, jealousy-related, or that you feel it's adulterous, it triggers your ick reflex, or you just think it's too fucking absurd to be sexual—and then make the effort to understand a little bit more about porn, and what it really means to your man. In our survey, a whopping 88 percent of male respondents said they at least sometimes use video pornography when masturbating. And 26 percent of these guys told us that their partners don't know about it! If you do harbor negative feelings toward porn, we have some interesting news for you: It turns out most men are smarter about porn than we think. Buckle up and read on!

DOES MODERN PORN MESS WITH YOUR GUY'S EXPECTATIONS OF SEX?

The pessimist in every woman assumes that porn fills men's minds with all kinds of strange, perverted, sexist ideas about the feminine half of the species and about sex in general. However, a great number of the men we interviewed told us that it doesn't alter their expectations at all. Says Ray, a 30-something customer service rep, "I think of porn as a fantasy world, like comics. People don't usually do those things. And most of the things I masturbate to I wouldn't want to try in real life anyway."

Says Greg, a 34-year-old veterinarian, "A lot of the things that I absolutely love in porn just don't translate to my real-life attractions. For example, huge tits are awesome in porn, but in real life, I love the small ones."

Tim, a 20-something Web designer put it more succinctly: "Porn is like the circus." In other words, it's fun to be a spectator, but he doesn't really want to be the man who rides around on a unicycle.

A healthy man will look at pornography as fantasy. Its purpose is to *supplement* his sex life and masturbatory practices. It should never be a substitute for the intimacy of having a real partner, and many men, especially those with at least some sexual experience, know this. That said, don't be surprised at the number of times your guy might look at video porn. Of the men we interviewed who were in healthy relationships, some reported looking at porn a few times a month, some do it a couple of times a week, and some, as Grammy nominee Brian McKnight joked on the 2005 "Boys Will be Boys" episode of *Oprah*, do it as often as once an hour (talk about a fast Internet connection!).

PORNO PITFALLS

Although pornography certainly has its place in healthy sex fantasy, there are times when it can cause issues. Some of the more common problems it can produce are detailed in the following.

SIZE OBSESSION

You've probably heard of the 1970s porn star John Holmes who sported a 10-inch (25.4 cm) woody, or the contemporary star Ron Jeremy who protrudes at a lengthy 9.75 inches (24.76 cm). These are just the more famous big dicks that have come on-screen over the years. Sixty percent of our real-life men reported having a 6-inch (15.24 cm) cock or smaller, which is at least 4 inches (10.16 cm) shy of the monster dicks depicted in porn. The problem occurs when our lovely, normal-sized men get it in their little heads that they should have bigger heads.

Next time your guy starts comparing his rod with Ron Jeremy's or any of those guys,' remind him that in addition to their above-average endowment (which is what got them the job in the first place), many male porn stars do things that trick viewers into believing their penises are larger than life.

Tips on What to Tell Your Man

- In mainstream porn, sex scenes usually involve petite women who automatically make the penis look bigger.
- Camera angles and close-ups eliminate perspective so that penises parade across the screen like Chinese dragons on New Year's Eve.
- Porn stars often shave or clip their pubic hair, which makes the shaft seem larger.
- Some stars even use penis pumps before a scene to temporarily enhance the size of their cocks.

PERFORMANCE PRESSURE

Another sad message that men may take away from porn is the impression that they should embody the lean, mean, fucking machines they see on the screen (or they may think *you* expect it). Although pornography may eliminate performance pressure for men while they are masturbating, it can have the opposite effect in the bedroom. Some men may expect they should be able keep a raging hard-on for hours at a time.

Gently remind your guy that several tricks are used to keep these porn stars going long and strong.

Tips on What to Tell Your Man

- Porn producers use sophisticated methods, including editing tricks, to prolong scenes. For example, often the same three-minute scene is repeated over and over again, from different angles, so that it seems there is a lot more in-and-out action than there really is.
- The director may cut the cameras off for a long break so that the actor can rejuvenate his boner off camera and get right back into the action when he's ready.
- Porn stars employ the use of ED drugs, including Viagra and Cialis. The latest trick is the use of a relatively new drug called Caverject that is injected via a needle and syringe into the base of the penis (it's not typically used outside of porn, as it hasn't been approved by the FDA yet).

All of this adds up to a very spectacular performance of erectile prowess. As Dr. Jenni says, "Remind your lover that real-life sex should be about *pleasure*, not performance." There is no need for him to try to live up to the ways of the porn star. As long as he is pleasing you, he is doing great.

HE EXPECTS YOU TO BEAR A BARE PUSSY

In the early days of porn, the bush was big. Women went au natural and nobody had a problem with that. But as pornography transitioned from the expression of a social movement into a lucrative enterprise, it became about getting the "better shot." Women's hair was removed for better visual access to the in-and-out action.

The gorgeous Marilyn Chambers (best known for her role in *Behind the Green Door*) was one of the first adult actresses to sport this sleek, new look. Now it has become such an ingrained aesthetic in our culture that women collectively spend millions of dollars a year on pubic hair removal!

Tips on What You Can Do

- Weigh your options and stand your ground. If you do remove your hair, it can enhance the sexual sensations during oral sex and intercourse for both partners.
- If you decide you want to keep what nature gave you, take heart in the knowledge that many men are starting to turn away from the bare look. "I've had a ton of women coming in saying that want to at least leave a triangle or a strip because their lovers actually like some hair," says Tammy, a 32-year-old body waxer.
- Remember, in the end, it's your body and your choice.

PORN BECOMES A COMPULSION

Porn is like junk food: It's nice for a sugary or salty snack, but it shouldn't be the sole source of sustenance. Unfortunately, some men become obsessed with pornography and it interferes with their relationships. Dr. Jenni says that if a man can go three full days without viewing porn, he's doing just fine. But if he can't, he should try to determine where this compulsion is coming from and perhaps consult a professional for help. Note that we're talking about the compulsion, not the practice. Your man may view porn every day, and if he does, that doesn't mean you should sound the alarm and alert the sexual deviance police that your man has a problem. The problem occurs when he psychologically can't go three days without viewing it.

Tips on What You Can Do

If you're worried that he's becoming compulsive, ask him nicely to take a rest for a little while. If he can and does, he's fine. In fact, count yourself lucky: You have a man with a healthy sexual appetite, and who graciously accommodates your wishes when you ask nicely! If he can't put it to rest, you may want to seek help from a sex therapist.

HE EXPECTS YOU TO FUCK LIKE A STARLET

A man who's relatively inexperienced with real women and real sex may expect his partner to act like a porn star. This means that he thinks she should be able to orgasm, loudly and theatrically, in minutes, always desire anal and oral sex, have big fake boobs, and enjoy cum dripping down her face.

> ### Dr. Glenda says:
>
> "Julia Roberts's films have done more damage to the status of women than all
> of the suck-and-fuck films ever made. Think of all of those romantic comedies that
> have women pursuing one man and giving up aspects of themselves to be with him."

Tips on What You Can Do

If you're up for any of this, more power to you, but if you're not, don't be afraid to just be yourself in bed. Taking the time to teach him how to be your best lover will also teach him that comparing real women to porn stars is like comparing flesh to jelly dildos.

PORNO PERKS

If you are both healthy and not suffering from porno pitfalls, you can use these naughty films as a way to add a whole new dimension to your sex life.

PORNOGRAPHY AS SEX EDUCATION
(Even Better Than That Reproductive Film They Showed You in Middle School)

Dr. Jenni tells us that, when used correctly, pornography can do wonders for one's sex life. It offers close-ups of genital anatomy in action, and it gives us possibilities in the sack that defy conventional wisdom—information that you'll likely not find anywhere else. Obviously, your mom, priest, or teacher will never discuss possible positions for three-ways, give you tips on how to wield a spanking crop, or show you what it looks like to deep throat a penis.

INSPIRATION FOR THE BEDROOM

Pornography can bring new and exciting ideas about positions and scenarios that you can actually use in your playtime. Maybe your man never knew that you were into spanking, double penetration, or the *Kama Sutra*. Choose a film that reflects your deepest desires and suggest that the two of you act out some of the scenarios together. Even simply copying some of the sex positions that the porn stars show on camera can be a titillating adventure. Don't worry if you don't pull it off, though, because what the porn stars don't know is that laughter definitely has its place in great sex.

SUGGESTED PORN-VIEWING LIST

If you are a porn novice, here are our favorite feel-good producers:

- Candida Royalle. This producer is known for weaving interesting and smart plotlines into gorgeous sex scenes. The men are equally as beautiful as the women, and the women experience sexual power and real orgasms. www.candidaroyalle.com

- Tristan Taormino. Taormino's *Chemistry* series includes real chemistry between porn actors and shows honest female orgasms. Taormino highlights safe, pleasurable anal sex, and some of her films feature incredible orgy scenes. www.puckerup.com

- Cinema Erotique. Cherry Chapman creates sensual, sexy, European-style pornography with fun plots, interesting camera work, and natural women. www.cinemaerotique.com

"PERVERTS" UNITE!

Pornography can reassure you that you're not the only one who gets a little freaky-deaky in the sack. It can be nice to know that you aren't the only person in the world who enjoys anal, flogging, bondage, rimming, blow jobs, group sex, or [insert your fantasy here]. Especially for individuals who have imaginative sexual desires (read: not vanilla), it's nice to see images of your deepest fantasies depicted on screen. You are not alone.

DEALING WITH CULTURAL, SOCIETAL, AND RELIGIOUS TABOOS

If you've ever been with a man who displayed guilt, degradation, or shame in his bedroom behavior, you've likely witnessed the manifestation of a cultural, societal, or religious taboo. These are behaviors that were taught and absorbed when your lover was but a young boy and stem from a variety of influential sources, including parents, family, church, friends, and school.

ANAL SEX IS WRONG, DIRTY, AND/OR GAY

In a fanatical sermon given by extremist Kansas Baptist pastor Fred Phelps, he said, "There's something about anal copulating that just drains the cells out of the brain."[40] Negative views on anal pleasure have been echoed in different ways across our culture. Even the significantly less conservative Dr. Drew Pinsky (of the popular radio sex show *Loveline*) frequently speaks against anal sex, often implying that it is a dirty and dangerous practice and suggesting that the anus is designed to be exit only. Additionally, because anal sex is a common method of intercourse in the gay community, many homophobic men have taken the stance that the act (especially if on the receiving end of a finger or dildo) is "gay."

So is anal sex dirty and dangerous? The answer is a qualified no. Some people have the impression that anal sex is riskier than vaginal sex because the anal tissue is very thin and more prone to tearing than the vaginal tissue is (which means a higher rate of STI transmission). However, it is just as safe as vaginal intercourse if proper precautions are taken. Safer practices include using condoms, making sure the playground is clean, and using plenty of lube. And for those who argue that the anus will suffer damage and begin to leak after too much anal penetration, we counterargue that the sphincter is a muscle and muscles are made for stretching.

If you put a sex toy or finger in his ass and he enjoys it, does this mean that your guy might be gay? No, of course not! It just means that you are both expanding your sexual horizons and exploring one of the many other erogenous zones on his body besides his cock. Congratulations on breaking his exclusively dick-centric sexuality.

Read chapter 5, "Funky Butt Lovin' and the P-Spot," for more information on safe, fun anal play.

MEN WHO GO DOWN ARE PUSSIES OR UNMANLY (After All, You Are What You Eat, Right?)
In season one, episode nine of *The Sopranos*, it is discovered that Junior Soprano enjoys going down on his girlfriend, Roberta. When Bobbi learns of these predilections, Junior cautions him not to tell anyone, "because they think if you'll suck pussy, you'll suck anything . . . It's a sign of weakness. And possibly a sign that you're a *fanook*." Now, chances are, your man isn't involved in the Italian mafia (and he also isn't likely a *fanook*—Mafioso-speak for the derogatory term *fag*), but this doesn't necessarily mean that he's not suffering from a bit of machismo.

In some cases, his hesitation may just be a question of cleanliness; some men are more sensitive to the heady scent of pussy. If he's not into cheese, oysters, or olives, you may have one of these guys on your hands. The simple solution is, of course, to bathe thoroughly before pushing his head beneath the sheets (making sure you're shower-fresh is a common courtesy).

Otherwise, religious or cultural reasons are often the culprit behind his unwillingness to give you this most pleasurable of all pleasures. Several women have told us that they find that their African American lovers are less likely to give head than their white counterparts, as they've been taught that it's "unmanly." One Muslim man told us that he refuses to give head for religious reasons, saying that his father taught him that "it would be like eating pork, and that is also against my religion."

While some men will never change their viewpoint on this topic, others can be rehabilitated with the right coaching.

Tips on Luring Him to Lick

- Keep your pussy clean and inviting.
- If he enjoys receiving head (like most men do), ask him to 69.
- Try popping in a porn video that shows a couple really enjoying cunnilingus—just to show him the fun he is missing.

The good thing is that there are plenty of men who are more than happy to dive right between your legs and stay there for as long as you'll have them. So if worst comes to worst and you haven't yet committed to your tongue-shy tease, find a guy who's more compatible with your desires.

WOMEN WHO GO DOWN ARE "COCKSUCKERS" OR WHORES

In Spike Lee's 1999 film *Summer of Sam*, the main character, Vinny, played by John Leguizamo, can't allow his wife, Dionna, to go down on him, although he has no problem screwing plenty of other women upside down and sideways.

Although most men won't turn down a blow job from any woman (whether they love her or not), nine percent of the women we surveyed said that they'd been with men who told them they were dirty or whorish for giving head. Evidently, there are still some men who suffer from the

> *Dr Glenda says:*
>
> "The notion that women who give blow jobs are whores is left over from when it was actually true in U.S. culture. It used to be that if you wanted your dick sucked, you went to another dude or a hooker. Nice girls didn't do that."

antiquated notion that blow jobs are something that are given only by prostitutes or gay men. If your guy is one of these, it's really his loss. You can either work with him to figure out where this perception came from, or relax your jaw muscles and live with it. Or you can go find one of the millions of men who actually enjoy having his penis inside a woman's mouth.

Dr. Glenda credits William Masters and Virginia E. Johnson with the shift in the cultural psyche regarding cocksucking. In the extensive research for their book, *Human Sexual Response* (1966), Masters and Johnson determined that receiving oral sex seriously enhanced women's arousal and consequently that turnabout was fair play. They encouraged everyone to enjoy oral sex—man or woman, naughty or nice.

THE "MADONNA/WHORE" SYNDROME

Many men will say that they want "a lady in the streets and a freak between the sheets." Some of these men, however, will never give their women a chance to be both a lady and a freak, or express any of the other things she may want to manifest. For the man who has the Madonna/whore problem, these roles become mutually exclusive in his mind and can cause a lot of headaches for women. Women who are seen as wholesome may have a difficult time finding men who are willing to allow them to be sexually expressive, while women who are viewed as easy and overtly sexual can often have a hard time finding men who will appreciate them as whole people and potential partners.

Says Lucy, a 20-something student, "My boyfriend often told me that he thought I was too beautiful to engage in slutty sex acts. I think he was turned on by somewhat taboo acts (bondage, latex), and had a real Madonna/whore complex. He liked to believe that his girlfriend was too pure to do such dirty things."

You have to wonder about a guy who wants a wholesome relationship as well as a kinky, exciting sex life but who refuses to combine the two. This type of man probably has a hard time being honest with himself as well as with the woman in his life. David, a 39-year-old programmer, confesses, "I travel a lot for business, and I visit a strip club everywhere I go. I have to admit, I love strippers. My wife of seven years knows I've been, but doesn't know just how often I indulge. She asked me once if I would take her to a strip club and I refused. She's just too good for a place like that."

In a case like this, the problems are manyfold. David has placed his "good" wife in the Madonna box, while the strippers are the women with whom he "indulges." He compartmentalizes so well that his wife doesn't get to be a whole person in their marriage (even when she asks!), and likewise, he never shows her all the facets of who he is. How lonely for both of them!

So what's a girl to do? Obviously, we don't suggest that you change to fit into one box or another.

Tips for the Madonna

If you've been placed in the Madonna box, take small steps to insinuate your sexual freaky side into your nice girl life:

- If he thinks you're the best cook since his mother, cook up his favorite meal wearing only a thong.
- Does he always order that classy glass of chardonnay for you when you go out? Stop him midsentence and order yourself a dirty martini—stress the *dirrrty*.
- Does he brag to his friends about how fit you are because all of the yoga and Pilates you do? Switch it up and install a stripper pole.

Tips for the Whore

Likewise, if you're generally perceived as a wild girl and can't rid yourself of all of those "whore" expectations and limitations, let him know just how nice you are and how nicely you expect to be treated:

- Does he love how you always make the naughty and incredibly entertaining sexual jokes and innuendos when talking with him and his friends? Change it up with talk of the stock market, sports, and your favorite cooking show channel.
- Does he always ask you to wear that sexy, revealing black top? Get ready without him and wear the beautiful, warm sweater instead.
- And ladies, you can make it clear that you're not always at his beck and call for that booty call.

SEX GUILT

In season one, episode twelve of *Sex and the City*, Miranda breaks up with "Catholic Guy" when he insists on showering immediately after intercourse because he believes that sex is intrinsically dirty, both physically and morally. Sadly, there are still many people out there who suffer from severe sex guilt as a result of their religious, cultural, or moral upbringing. People who grew up being told that masturbating can cause hair to grow on their palms, acne, or blindness, or even worse, damn them for eternity, may still be carrying this type of sex guilt into their partner play.

Eleven percent of the women we surveyed reported that they'd been with a partner who experienced sex guilt. Some of the more common reasons for men feeling guilty about sex (excluding cheating) include the following:

- **"Shameful" sex acts (threesomes, anal sex, and bondage, oh my!).** Jack Morin, author of *The Erotic Mind* (1996), put it best when he wrote, "Anything that turns us off can potentially turn us on, and vice versa." The best way to handle guilt around shameful sex acts is to embrace the guilty pleasure that they bring. For example, it's actually much more fun to have sex outside for fear of getting caught. Take out that fear and you miss out on most of the fun! What about anal sex? Part of the excitement may be the idea that it's dirty and bad. Add a few spankings, and you've got yourself a guilty treat that burns more calories than you can eat in a fully loaded ice cream sundae. Help your partner to capitalize on the thrill of sex guilt by egging him on, "Oh, I love it when you lick my ass, you bad boy!"

- **Sex before marriage.** Your boyfriend may be dead serious when he says, "No rock, no cock," in which case you need to decide whether that's an acceptable relationship rule for you. But if he's just halfheartedly parroting lessons from long ago while his penis points at you like a divining rod, then maybe you can both enjoy the taste of the forbidden fruit that is premarital nookie.
- **Men who feel like they aren't pleasing their partners.** Surprisingly, the most common reason behind sex guilt, as discovered in our survey, came from men who came too quickly and didn't allow time for their partners to orgasm. This could be a sign that you aren't speaking up in bed and demanding more pleasure. The easiest way to ensure your orgasm is to not allow the sex act to escalate from zero to "holy shit I'm coming!" too quickly. If he can't please you, it's up to you to show him how. Break out the sex toys, make him go down on you, and start enforcing the all-important house rule: Ladies come first! For more tips on handling premature ejaculation, read chapter 8, "His Libido: Understanding your Hornball."
- **More serious issues.** If your man was the victim of sexual assault, an abusive upbringing, or any other insidious incidents that cause him to experience debilitating sex guilt, he should speak with a qualified therapist.

A GENTLEMAN COWBOY ON YOUR HANDS

In addition to the negative impressions that may shape your guy as a lover, he may also be, simply put, a gentleman. Most, if not all, men in our culture are raised with certain codes of conduct, and the most stringent of these codes is: Don't ever hurt a girl (or as cowboy legend Gene Autry says, "Respect women"). Overall, of course, this is a good principle to teach our men, but it may bring interesting consequences to the bedroom; your lover may have a strong aversion to indulging certain desires because he's afraid of breaking the ultimate man mandate.

The O&C survey revealed that many men are afraid of trying things such as anal sex, light spanking, or even role-playing because they don't want to hurt their partners. Jeff, a 37-year-old writer, says, "I am not into pain, and have a very, very hard time [inflicting] pain on my partner. I was once asked to 'rape' a lover, and I just could not be rough or painful enough—it goes against my being on how to treat a woman (any woman)."

So if, indeed, your own desires involve your lover serenading you with phrases such as "nasty bitch" and "dirty slut," or you're dreaming that he'll turn the canvas of your bum into a nice, stinging collage of pink handprints, the Cowboy Code of treating women with respect may turn into quite an obstacle for you. However, there are ways to work with your lover and let him know that what you're after is pleasure, which can come in many forms.

Tips on How to Handle Your Cowboy
- Remind him that your sex life and your waking life are two very different things. While you love and appreciate his kindness and respect out of the bed, you'd love and appreciate even more his sternness in the bed.
- Gratitude and praise. For every little swat he dishes to your backside, be sure to compliment him tenfold and positively reinforce him by doing something pleasing for him in return.
- Leave it be. Sometimes there is no hope of turning a gentleman into a fantasy-fulfilling machine. Times like this you've got to decide whether the man or the kink is more important.
- And ladies, any of the tips in chapter 10, "His Inner Beast: Bring Out the Sexual Wild Side of your Man," can be applied here as well.

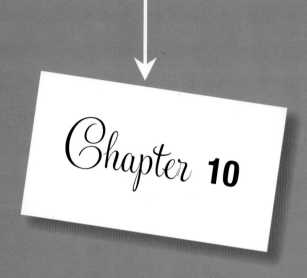

Chapter 10

HIS INNER BEAST: BRING OUT THE SEXUAL WILD SIDE OF YOUR MAN

WHEN WE THINK OF A MAN'S SEXUAL WILD SIDE, we can't help but think about the iconic children's classic *Where the Wild Things Are* by Maurice Sendak. The story is the perfect metaphor: Punished and sent to bed without supper, the child travels in his imaginary boat to an island "where the wild things are." When he first meets the wild things, they seem like toothy, drooling, snarling monsters. Some might say they are scary. However, the child in the story quickly learns how to play with the wild things, and they have a wonderfully wicked time together. The riotous and untamed night of fun ends with the perfect image: A large wild thing sleeping with a big peaceful grin on his face underneath a tree.

Think of this story in adult life. Most couples have the basics covered—they have a handful of tried-and-true techniques to get their partners off, whether it's a firm, light squeeze of the testes during oral sex, or that perfect position that guarantees mutual climax. However, at some point, most women feel that they are ready to take their sex lives past the basics and tap deeper into the sexual side of their partners. In other words, they are ready to set out in their imaginary boats and meet their man's inner wild thing.

This is an important journey in any intimate relationship, because it provides a more authentic connection to your partner and who he is as a lover and as a man. If the thought of your man's sexual wild side is a little intimidating, just think of the fun that Max had riding on the back of the biggest wild thing. And then remember the sweet, satisfied smile that the same wild thing wore as he slept at the end of the story. Now, don't you want to see that same smile on your man's grateful face?

JUST ASK

For some lucky gals, bringing out his sexual beast is simply a matter of asking. Statements like, "Tell me what you want me to do to you" and "Let's try something we've never done before" will inspire honest and enthusiastic answers and acts from your man. The question, "What is your deepest, most hidden fantasy, honey?" will surely bring out his true sexual beast. If your partner is one of these open and communicative types, then conversing with him is the best first step to meeting his inner wild thing. But keep in mind that the rest of the techniques in this chapter will work for you as well. There are many aspects of sexual enjoyment and experience that lie beyond the conscious threshold of dialogue.

BEYOND WORDS

As enlightened and aware as most modern men are, there is often still a communication gap between the genders, especially when it comes to sex. If you ask your partner, "What is your deepest, most hidden fantasy, honey?" and he answers, "To make love to you," you know you've got your work cut out for you.

Why is this? According to Ian Kerner, Ph.D., "Numerous studies, as well as my own clinical experience, support the fact that many individuals see their sexual fantasies in a somewhat negative light, and, thereby, repress them to varying degrees."[41]

It makes sense. Many of us are taught from a very young age that sex is dirty and that our own sexual impulses make us perverted. Whether we pick this information up from religious teachings, our parents, friends, or other social influences, we all receive some negative conditioning around sex. These negative messages may be the building blocks that make up the walls that keep your man's sexual beast imprisoned.

IMAGINATION AND CREATIVITY: NAVIGATING YOUR WAY TO WILD THING ISLAND

Creativity and imagination are essential tools when discovering and luring out his inner sexual beast. The goal is to set sail on your imaginary boat and find your way to his wild island so that the two of you can play in sexy abandon.

INDULGE IN A LITTLE NOOKIE OVER THE PHONE

Ladies, you have no idea how intimate or revealing articulating a sex act with your partner can be.

If you're new to phone sex, or a little shy, start out slow. Ask him to describe a sexy outfit he'd like to see you in. Goad him on with questions about which of your body parts he likes the most and why. If you're past the initial stages of shy phone sex, ask him to describe, step-by-step, what he would do to you if you were to wear that sexy outfit. Don't let him gloss over the foreplay or skimp out on using the dirty words. You'll be surprised by what you'll learn when he vocally expresses what he notices about you and what he loves to do with you.

Says Regina, a 47-year-old human resources manager, "I had to travel a lot last year for work, and my husband and I started to experiment with phone sex to keep our sex life active and interesting. One night, he described how he loves to kiss the hollow of my neck while he slides his fingers inside me. He said, 'I love it because when I glance down, I can see your toes curling, and I know I'm driving you wild.' I had no idea that my toes curled when I was turned on—and even less of an idea that he paid attention! After fifteen years of marriage, this was a very sweet, and very hot, revelation."

NAUGHTY STORIES ARE YOUR FRIENDS

Erotica is one creative avenue to use that will lead you to his inner desires and fantasies. Encourage him to read erotica, either in book format or online, and then ask him to share his favorite stories with you. If your man is a creative-type, ask him to write you an erotic short story. The two of you can also practice reading short stories to one another before bed. All of these activities give him a means to indirectly (or directly) express inner fantasies, and you can glean a lot of information from what he chooses to read or write. Moreover, reading and writing erotica is an arousing activity. We guarantee that not only will you learn something about his wild side, but doing these exercises will, simply put, turn you both on.

EMBRACE PORNOGRAPHY

Video porn is another avenue that can be used in a similar way, and requesting to watch it together is a good way to gain access to some of his inner fantasies. If you're not quite ready to delve into his long-enjoyed collection, you may want to purchase a DVD yourself and surprise him, or better yet, pick out a video together. Paying attention to what scenes he responds to in the films and, even more important, how he responds, will help you unveil his sexual wild side.

An important note on pornography if you are planning to sail your boat in this direction: Be prepared to discover that your partner may enjoy watching women who look or act wholly different from you. This does not mean that he's not attracted to you; it simply means that he's human and enjoys variety in his fantasy life (don't we all?). The important thing to remember as you explore his pornographic tastes (and anything else you explore in your quest to find his wild side) is to keep an open mind. Sexual curiosities, propensities, fetishes, and desires can be incredibly varied within one individual. Thank goodness this is so, because in the end, that's what keeps our sex lives interesting and our relationships strong.

PLAY DATES AT ADULT TOY STORES

Adult toy stores and fetish stores provide a playful environment in which to observe the behavior of your man's inner wild thing. On your next date night, take him out for a glass of wine and then go to the local sex shop. Allow him to take the lead and watch where he goes in the store, what he looks at, what he picks up, and where his eyes dart. Take mental notes; they will provide great ideas for you for later experimentation. Better yet, experiment tonight: Make a purchase together and use it as soon as you get home.

GIVE HIM SPECIFICS

Let's face it, ladies: Men are fixers and like to deal in specifics. Even the most uncommunicative guy can answer a detail-oriented question—especially if you put it in a "I have a problem that needs to be solved" sort of way. Just as you might ask him, "Honey, what kind of tool should I use to tighten this screw? The wrench or the screwdriver?" feel free to ask him, "Honey, what kind of tool should I use in our next screw session? The blindfold or the flogger?" You get the picture. Ask him if there's a toy or prop he'd like to use (a rope, a feather, hot wax, etc.), and then indulge him.

Tips on Being Sexually Specific

- Ask him what sexy garment he'd like to see you wear.
- Give him two options on lingerie: black and vinyl, or white and lacey.
- Have him choose the location of your next sexual encounter (i.e., the bathtub, the kitchen counter, the backseat of the car).
- If you get invited to a sex-toy party, or are heading to the local adult toy store, ask him for his wish list.

Keep the questions simple and specific, and you may get information out of him yet!

CONFIDENCE: THE TEETH AND CLAWS OF THE BEAST

Let us remind you of a great scene in the 1996 film *Swingers*. Trent Walker (played by Vince Vaughn—now there's one sexy beast!) is talking to Mike Peters (played by Jon Favreau) and likens Mike to a bear that should see women as his prey—namely bunnies. Trent holds his fingers up like claws and, wild-eyed, exclaims:

> *"You got these fuckin' claws, and these fangs, man. And you're looking at your claws and you're looking at your fangs. And you're thinking to yourself, you don't know what to do, man. 'I don't know how to kill the bunny.' With this [Trent holds his clawed fingers up to demonstrate], you don't know how to kill the bunny, do you know what I mean?"*

The entire point that Trent is trying to make is that when it comes to women (and sex), confidence is key. All men have the claws and the fangs—in other words, they are, in part, a sexual beast—but they may lack the confidence to let that beast loose. Confidence imbues men with a sense of sexual power; it makes them feel attractive and more sexually open. It helps them to feel that they have prowess in the bedroom. It makes them more experimental and better lovers. If you nurture your lover's sense of confidence, he will be more inclined to bare those sexy teeth and claws and let his inner wild thing come out to play. Don't worry—he won't bite you, unless you ask.

BUTTER HIM UP

Women aren't the only ones who love a compliment. In the context of the everyday, try to find ways to authentically compliment your lover. When he gets out of the shower, tell him how nice he looks in the nude. When he gets ready for work, tell him how sexy he looks in a suit. If he's just sitting in front of the TV drinking a beer, let him know how much you enjoy being around him when he's relaxed. The key is to connect compliments with the idea of sex, or his sexuality, in some way—a surefire way to help nurture his confidence.

POSITIVE REINFORCEMENT

It's a technique used to train animals of all types, from puppies to dolphins. The basic concept is simple: Positively reinforce or reward the behavior you like, and simply don't respond to the behavior that you don't like. This will both help build his confidence and condition him to be a better lover for you.

So if you like the way he swirls his tongue around your nipple, let him know! Tell him how good it feels, arch your back, moan, grasp his shoulders—whatever you can do to enthusiastically communicate that he's doing it just right.

POSITIVE REINFORCEMENT, ACCORDING TO THE SSPCA[42]

HINT: If it works for your pet, it will work for your guy.

• Positive reinforcement is the presentation of something pleasant or rewarding immediately following a behavior. It makes that behavior more likely to occur in the future and is one of the most powerful tools for shaping or changing your pet's behavior.

• Correct timing is essential when using positive reinforcement. The reward must occur immediately, or your pet may not associate it with the proper action. For example, if you have your dog sit but reward him after he's already stood up again, he'll think he's being rewarded for standing up.

• Consistency is also essential.

On the flip side, when he moves on to do something you may not be a fan of, please don't ruin the mood by telling him right then and there that you hate what he's doing. This is called negative reinforcement and is counterproductive. It engenders bad feelings all around and may in fact kill the sexual mood altogether. Your simple silence or lack of response should be information enough for him. If he continues to do something that you're just not too keen on, offer an alternative. If he is licking your belly and you'd rather him lick something else, suggestively whisper something like, "Oh baby, I love the way your tongue feels on my inner thigh."

The key is to always keep your reactions and vocal suggestions positive. And ladies, do so with enthusiasm. Make it clear when he does something right, and he will not only seek to do more right more often, but he will do so with confidence.

THE BEAST WITH TWO BACKS (OR, IT TAKES TWO TO TANGO)

There may be several poetic reasons why William Shakespeare referred to sex as "the beast with two backs." For our conversation, it's an important image, because it signifies that in sex, two people join to become one and—strikingly—it's not one person, but one beast. The point, ladies, is that to truly draw out the sexual beast in your man, you must show him your own sexual beast. It takes the trust and magic of two to make the wild tango work.

KEEP HIM "IN THE KNOW" ABOUT WHAT TURNS YOU ON

Many of the suggestions made for bringing out his sexual beast can be tweaked just a little and used to show him your sexual beast. Tools such as erotica and pornography can be your messenger boys, as well. Says Sarah, a 27-year-old writer, "I've been jonesin' for a good spanking, but my boyfriend just wasn't getting it. I gave him an anthology of BDSM short stories to read, and let's just say he's not only taken the hint, but he's taken to spanking like a fish to water!"

Other basics include sharing your own fantasies during a session of phone sex or introducing your own props or toys to the bedroom in a playful way. (Let's try to stay away from pulling out the huge dildo and telling him you'd rather fuck the toy than him—not a good confidence booster for the beast you're trying to nurture.) You get the picture.

WRITE YOUR OWN SEX MANUAL

This is an invaluable tool for you and your man in the bedroom. Writing a sex manual all about yourself and giving it to your man will not only make him feel empowered as a lover (think of it as his very own "claw and tooth" sharpener), but it will also ensure that you get the things you need from your lover.

Catherine, a 30-something public relations manager, says, "I created my own illustrated sex manual for my boyfriend, with tips on how and when to pull my hair, how much pressure to apply during oral sex, and what to do if I look bored. I didn't know it was such a hit until I was making his bed one day and found it tucked under his mattress in a spot that was within easy reach for him. It looked very well-read."

Your own personal sex manual can be written and rewritten as your sex life evolves. And not only is it educational for him, but you may also discover some fun things about yourself! See chapter 12, "Go Forth and F*CK," for your very own personal sex manual.

As you might gather, ladies, the creative ways you can discover and indulge your lover's sexual wild beast are endless. However you choose to navigate your way to his sexy wild island, be ready for some skips, bumps, a few big waves, and even an unexpected wayward wind. After all, half of the fun is in the journey, and finding your very own wild thing will be well worth it.

MEN REVEAL SOME OF THEIR TOP, UNFULFILLED FANTASIES

- "To get picked up in a bar!"
- "Swinging with other bisexual, married couples."
- "Sex on the beach."
- "To have my very own sex slave."
- "Observing lesbian sex."
- "To be with an older woman."
- "Watching a woman masturbate from start to finish."
- "I'd like to have vigorous, passionate sex outside, in the middle of a violent thunderstorm."
- "I want to be arse fucked by a woman."
- "To have my wife swallow me."
- "To have sex on a motorcycle at 80 mph."
- "To wake up to an unsolicited blow job."
- And of course, the "classic" male fantasy of sex with multiple partners got many a mention.

As you can see, some of these fantasies are wild and even unsafe (a motorcycle at 80 mph? We don't think so!), while others are downright simple (just suck it up and swallow it already). But whether cute or crazy, fantasy is just that—fantasy. As adults, we all know that some of it may be actualized one day, while the rest will remain fodder for dreams or a good masturbatory session! The important thing is to be able to talk about fantasy and embrace your lover's sexual imaginings.

IS HE A PERVERT?

Some people are afraid of exploring fantasy because they don't want to examine their own desires or those of their partners. In fact, many sexual predilections that don't fit "the norm" may be seen as being dangerous or perverted. However, when you attempt to delve deeper into someone's wild sexual nature, it's quintessentially important to keep an open mind. Remember that fantasy is born of the imagination, and if you listen with an open heart when he tells you he wants to fuck you while he wears your pantyhose, he may return the favor when it comes to reacting to your own dirty little desire, whatever that may be.

There are many layers to fantasy and many ways to indulge in them. Think of fantasy as a rainbow of possibilities.

At one end of the rainbow is full, physical indulgence—your pot of gold, if you will. For example, if your lover confesses that he fantasizes about going down on you while some strange man comes in and takes him anally, and you think this is just the best thing since ribbed condoms, then by all means, make a play date!

Along the arc of the rainbow, where the colors shimmer and blend, is exploring the fantasy through other erotic activities, such as writing or reading stories or watching a video together. For example, if your partner says he wants to have wild crazy sex with eight women at the same time, and that's just not your bag, you can always ask him to write it out for you in short story form. Or you can buy him a naughty DVD featuring such a scenario and watch it together.

And at the far end of the rainbow, that end that you can never find, is the "no-fly zone." This, of course, is reserved for fantasies of which you want no part. A good solution for dealing with this type of fantasy would be to say, "No, thank you, but please incorporate it into your masturbatory life as much as you please." For example, if your sweetie wants, more than anything, for you to pee on his face, and your reaction is the inability to even look him in the eye for a few minutes after this admission, let alone contemplate acting it out, it's okay to the draw the line. Tell him that you're just not interested, but if he wants to fantasize about this during his private time, he should go for it. This will make your own desires clear, while keeping the fantasy conversation positive for both of you.

The thing to keep in mind is that, while exploring fantasy and encouraging his wild sexual side to come out, it's not necessary to physically act on each and every desire. In fact, there may be fantasies that he actually doesn't want to realize; he just likes to talk about them. Moreover, bringing his every whim to life may actually be impossible.

Take, for example, Tanner, 28, a real estate developer, whose top three fantasies are as follows (in no particular order):

1. "Have a girl choke me until I pass out."

2. "Have a hot-ass waitress give me 'that look,' and we end up fucking in the janitor's closet."

3. "A school bus full of eighteen-year-old girls and they all think I'm the Messiah."

Tanner is happily dating a doctor and has shared fantasy number one with her in the hopes that she will not only indulge him, but will also have the medical expertise not to kill him in the process. He confesses that he's actually done fantasy number two and still dreams about it, but won't act on it now that he's in a relationship. And fantasy number three is, he admits, hilariously impossible—"but a guy can dream, can't he?"

And yes, that's the point: Fantasy feeds desire, whether it is ever acted on or not. The fuller your lover's fantasy life is and the more you encourage him to explore and share it, the better your sex life will be.

FETISHES VERSUS KINKS

In your quest to better understand your kinkster, it's best to understand the difference between a fetish and a kink.

FETISHES

Way back in the seventeenth century, the word *fetish* was used to describe objects with magical powers. These were talismans and charms that inspired reverence in the person who carried or looked upon them. Today, the word has evolved to relate to objects that inspire the "magical" feelings of arousal.

Technically speaking, a fetish is a reliance on a prop, body part, or scene to get sexually aroused or get off sexually. So if your lover indeed has a foot fetish, then feet are a necessary, central element to his sex life; he in fact will need to view, touch, caress, lick, or fantasize about feet to become aroused or achieve ejaculation. And with a real fetish, the person will have a sexual reaction to the object of his fetish even in nonsexual situations. For example, the man with a foot fetish could easily see a pair of comely feet standing in line at the gas station and grow an immediate erection, right there and then, with no other stimulation.

The sad thing about real fetishes is that, unless a lover magically shares the matching reciprocal fetish (i.e., a man with a foot fetish would need someone who must have her feet worshipped so she can orgasm), it can feel as if the fetishist is actually only turned on by the object of his fetish, and not his lover.

So where do fetishes originate? Psychologists say that a fetish is part of a person's sexual template and that it arises from a combination of social, psychological, and life experiences. In other words, they don't really know.

The good news is, in today's medical field, fetishism is viewed as normal variation in human sexuality, and it is considered unobjectionable as long as the parties involved feel comfortable.

KINKS

In the seventeenth century, the word *kink* was used as a nautical term to describe a twist in a rope. Today, it's commonly used to describe twisted sexual behavior. Think of kink, then, as an interest in or proclivity toward a prop, body part, or scene that lies outside of what is considered "normal" sexual behavior. If your lover simply adores your feet and likes to suck your toes as part of your sex play, but it's not necessary for his arousal or ejaculation, then he's just kinky. In actuality, the majority of people out there have kinks, not fetishes.

Dr. Jenni says:

"Fetishes are ingrained in one's innate sexual template and emerge more strongly should the external environment create a permissible (or sometimes not so permissible) situation to do so. Those with a true fetish *need* the desired object to become aroused. That said, shoes are cultural constructs. I mean, what did a shoe fetish look like 2000 years ago?"

UNUSUALLY COMMON FETISHES AND FANTASIES

Now that we've established that fantasy is a key player in facilitating a healthy sex life, it's time to educate yourself about some of the sexual predilections you might encounter. Even though they may seem unusual, these desires are more common than you might think.

Men who participated in the O&C sex survey revealed varied interests in all types of kinks and fetishes. Many men surveyed had experience with BDSM, but interestingly, most were *curious* about exploring swinging.

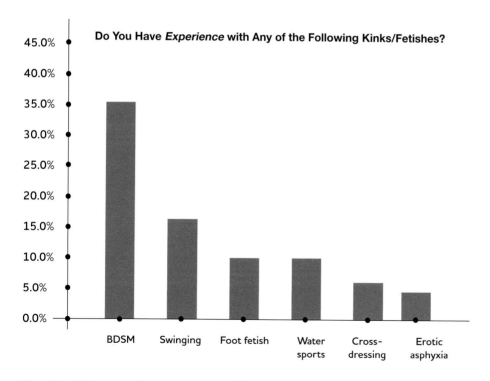

Do You Have *Experience* with Any of the Following Kinks/Fetishes?

More then 35 percent of men we surveyed said they have experience with BDSM.

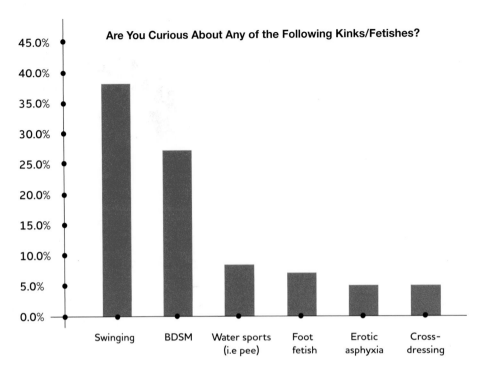

Are You Curious About Any of the Following Kinks/Fetishes?

45.0%	
40.0%	
35.0%	
30.0%	
25.0%	
20.0%	
15.0%	
10.0%	
5.0%	
0.0%	

Swinging | BDSM | Water sports (i.e pee) | Foot fetish | Erotic asphyxia | Cross-dressing

Nearly 40 percent of the men we surveyed are curious about swinging.

Other interests that received honorable mention include sex in public, pantyhose fetishes, voyeurism, knife play, and a desire to be anally penetrated by a woman with a strap-on.

IF YOUR GUY IS INTO SPANKINGS, BONDAGE, AND NIPPLE CLAMPS . . .

Then your guy is into BDSM, which stands for *bondage, domination, submission, and sadomasochism.* BDSM is a monster of a term because it encompasses both fetishes and kink. Moreover, it can either be simply a "tourist attraction," or it can be a way of life and can even be considered a sexual identity.

At heart, BDSM is about consensual power play; there is always a dominant partner and a submissive partner. Sometimes the partner's roles are static, but other times they will switch depending on the situation. Often, BDSM involves elaborate scenes, roles, and props that combine with the power play.

Power play includes humiliation games. For example, one partner may require the other to prance about like a pony wearing nothing but a butt plug. It also includes mild to severe infliction of physical torment by use of nipple clamps, spankings, floggings, and more. But mostly, it's about psychological control. For the dominant, this means being in control and being given permission to manipulate a person sexually to match his or her every desire. For the submissive, it's about relinquishing control and letting the dominant take the reins for a while. While on the surface, it would appear that the dominant partner has the upper hand, it's actually the submissive who sets the guidelines and rules of the game play.

Deanna, a professional artist and a 49-year-old lifestyle submissive, describes the experience: "It's not all about sex; it's a power exchange. There is power in being a sub. Very few women will go to the extremes that I do; it makes me feel secure in my relationship, complete, and irreplaceable."

Her husband Max, 53, agrees. "I've never been in a relationship with a woman like Deanna. We have an understanding that she's submissive to my every desire in the bedroom. The only boundary we have is that there are no boundaries, and she trusts me with that. In turn, I am more than happy to submit to her needs outside the bedroom."

BDSM lifestylers like Max and Deanna choose to remain "closeted" and keep their sexual identity a complete secret, carefully constructing a pristinely normal facade around their unusual sex lives. Singles and couples living the lifestyle may seek out like-minded individuals and frequent underground BDSM clubs or dungeons where they can act out their chosen scenarios in an understanding and titillating environment. Yet others may openly bring the domination/submission element into facets of their lives outside of the bedroom and the dungeon, turning the submissive partner into a 24/7 slave.

People who are considered "tourists" may try out BDSM-type scenarios such as using light bondage and candle wax, and they may even visit BDSM clubs to observe and arouse, but they typically only use these ideas to spice up a generally vanilla sex life.

IF YOUR GUY HAS A THING FOR YOUR TOES OR ARMPITS . . .

Then he's got a fetish or kink for parts of your body (also known as partialism). Remember season two, episode twenty-four of *Sex and the City* wherein Charlotte kept scoring awesome new shoes because a particular shoe salesman got off from placing the shoes on her feet? That, ladies, was a prime example of a foot fetish. He literally reached orgasm through the experience of touching and manipulating her feet. Once you get the image of his creepy O face out of your mind, let us remind you that actual body part fetishes (and fetishes in general) are very rare. On the flip side, it could be argued that almost every man has some kinky desire for at least one female body part—otherwise, why the question, "Are you an ass-man, a legs-man, or a boobs-man?" The fact that your lover may find your feet, neck, or even armpits (yes, we did talk to one man who just loved the armpits) to be the sexiest part of your body just means that he's not your typical guy. How refreshing!

IF YOUR GUY JUST CAN'T STOP TOUCHING YOUR PANTYHOSE . . .

Then he's got a kink or fetish for objects. "My husband loves to rip my pantyhose off of me before we have sex. He says the sound and feel of ripping the fabric is a real turn-on for him," says Mary, 38, a stay-at-home mom.

What Mary is describing here is one kinky guy. Her husband has a sexual affection for ripping pantyhose off of her; the pantyhose is the kinky part, but the fact that he needs his wife for the act makes it a kink and not a fetish. If, however, she starts finding ripped pantyhose in the tool shed or laying beside his weight machine, then she'll know that the ripping of the pantyhose is the sexual act for him and she has a fetishist on her hands.

Kinky affection for objects, especially clothing, can actually be a fun asset in the bedroom. When a man has a kinky thing for seeing you in a certain garment, he's actually enjoying your body as well as the object—it's *you* in that hat or in that fabulous pair of Jimmy Choos that drives him wild; without you, the objects are simply clothes that have no sexual weight for him. Having a clothing kinkster for a lover could be a little slice of heaven. After all, what girl doesn't like to play dress-up once in a while?

IF YOUR GUY WANTS TO BE BREATHLESS WHEN HE EJACULATES . . .

Then he's into erotic asphyxia (EA), otherwise known as asphyxiophilia, or breath play. EA, which has been documented as a practice since the 1600s, is the act of cutting off the air supply (or the blood flow, which produces the same result) during sex or masturbation. EA is an incredibly dangerous practice, as illustrated by David Carradine's alleged cause of death in 2009; between five hundred and a thousand deaths per year are attributed to EA, but experts agree this number is most likely inaccurately low, because so many of these deaths are labeled suicides rather than accidental deaths due to autoerotic asphyxiation (when one does it during masturbation).

So what's the appeal? Cutting off the blood flow to the brain during arousal and orgasm induces what is called cerebral anoxia, a state in which oxygen is deficient in the brain tissue. Oxygen deficiency is thought to intensify sensations and produce feelings of exhilaration or giddiness. Also, many people who practice EA, or who want to, have a strong masochistic drive.

While we believe it's incredibly important to keep an open mind regarding all things sexual, we do advise you stay clear of EA. Aside from the oh-so-huge disaster it would be to accidentally kill your lover by indulging him a fantasy, there's also a strong chance that you could simply turn him into a vegetable. The brain cannot withstand oxygen deficiency for more than a few minutes before permanent brain damage sets in. Let's face it ladies, a brain-dead lover is just not sexy (even if you are into jocks).

IF YOUR GUY LOVES PLAYING WITH PEE . . .

He's into water sports. No, we're not talking surfing here. Water sports and golden showers are both nice ways of summing up the act of including piss in your sex play.

Also know as urolagnia, this kind of play is a turn-on for its practitioners for a variety of reasons, which are emotional, psychological, and physical. The ideas that pee is "dirty" and that including it in sex is "bad" really get some people going; the shame factor is an arousing aspect of the play. Other people feel that letting go in every way, including with their bladders, simply increases intimacy and thus enhances their sexual relationship. And for some women, indulging in pee play is an extension of the physical reality that a semifull or full bladder often increases vaginal sensitivity during sex.

If you are curious about golden showers or you're considering indulging your lover, here are a few facts that will make you feel warm and cozy: First, urine is 95 percent water, 2.5 percent salt and other minerals, and 2.5 percent urea—which is why some people have been known to drink it and survive when no other water sources are available. Second, urine is very sterile—clean enough and antiseptic enough to be used to clean wounds, should modern medicine ever fail us. The truth is, urine is a benign substance when it comes from a healthy individual who drinks plenty of water. Just be sure to pass on the asparagus.

IF YOUR GUY WEARS FRILLY LINGERIE . . .

Then he's into cross-dressing. What does it mean when he wants to wear your lingerie? Is he transgendered? Is he gay? Will he want to go to your neighbor's dinner party dressed in a spicy little red number?

ASSUME THE GOLDEN SHOWER POSITION

Classic urolagnia positions run the gamut of possibility. Some of the more famous positions are:

- The woman sits on top of the man's penis in cowgirl position, but instead of actually fucking him, she pees. (Men who enjoy this particular water sport often report immediate orgasms.)

- The man gives the woman (who has an unbelievably full bladder—she's been saving up for this special occasion) oral sex and she lets go and pees only when she cannot possibly hold it any longer, or when she orgasms. The man is supposed to continue licking her through her pee until she is finished.

- The man stands over the woman (with a semiflaccid or flaccid penis, since it's impossible for him to pee with a raging hard-on) and pees directly on her clitoris. She can masturbate as he does this.

- The woman squats over the man and gives him a nice, old-fashioned hand job. However, there's a twist: When he's ready to come, he lets her know, and she pees forcefully on his cock as he orgasms.

The answers are no, no, and probably not (well, he may want to, but he probably won't go through with it). The truth is, most cross-dressing men (CDs) are straight and usually married. According to Paul Joannides, most cross-dressers actually have stereotypically "male" jobs, such as firemen, baseball players, mechanics, executives, and policemen. In other words, they are übermasculine, and they only indulge their feminine side by putting on those pretty panties.[43]

If you catch your manly man with his hand in your underwear drawer, be gentle. There is such a stigma against straight, "normal" men wearing women's clothing, and he's most likely been deathly afraid of you finding out. He is getting sexual stimulation by identifying with women, but he's identified as a straight male. In other words, he still wants to ravish your beautiful body, he may just want to do it now and again wearing his size 12 pink pumps.

IF YOUR GUY INSISTS ON INVITING NEW PARTNERS INTO THE RELATIONSHIP . . .

Then he's a swinger or a polyamorist. In our culture, it's the norm for people to seek out "the one," fall in love, get married, and live a monogamous lifestyle. However, this isn't the only relationship model out there, and many individuals opt for an alternative lifestyle. Swingers and polyamorists reject the notion of monogamy in favor of the idea that it's possible to enjoy healthy relationships with multiple sex and even multiple love partners.

While it's very common for men to eroticize the notion of having sex with two or more women at a time, this greatly differs from a swinging lifestyle. Swingers typically become very involved in communities of like-minded individuals. They often strike up deep and meaningful relationships with other couples and individuals who share this lifestyle. Some couples only engage in swinging with one other couple in the privacy of a home, and others go to swingers' parties or clubs, or even go to national swinging conventions! True swingers follow a very explicit code of conduct that involves respect and consensual interactions.

Sarah, a 61-year-old attorney, explains the dynamics of the swingers' club where she and her boyfriend are members: "The club we go to actually gives me a huge picture of all the varied ways people swing. It's a [heterosexual] couples only club, and single women are permitted. The number-one rule is to always ask permission, even before you kiss someone. The ages range from people in their thirties to people in their seventies. Most of the couples I've met there are married (to each other). Some of the couples arrive together but then don't see each other for the rest of the night; other couples have rules, such as only oral sex with others, no intercourse. One couple comes weekly but only has sex with each other. They dance and then go off to a room for sex. They like to be watched. Some couples come to meet another couple with whom they can develop a relationship outside of the club. Some women want to have sex with other women, and their partners are only too happy to watch."

Adds her boyfriend, Paul, 43, "There is only one private room—and no doors are ever locked. My favorite is the group room, referred to as the 'cluster-fuck!' One-ways, two-ways, three-ways! Anything goes in that room." The owners of the club frequented by Paul and Sarah say that when they polled their clientele, it was fifty-fifty between the male and female partners on whose idea it was to join the club in the first place.

If your guy puts the *grrr* in swin*ger*, baby, be prepared to share your modern-day Austin Powers!

OTHER KINKY ODDS AND ENDS . . .

If you were unfortunate enough to see the oh-so-icky online video "Two Girls, One Cup" (think poo in a cup), a turn-on to those who have coprophilia and get off on feces, then you know that there are at least a few more fetishes and kinks that we haven't touched on. Indeed, if you're a fan of *CSI*, then you already know about "furries" (people who enjoy dressing up in animal costumes to have sex) and adult babies and diaper lovers (need we say more?). The truth is, there are so many proclivities and sexual interests out there, it would be impossible to discuss all of them. If you can imagine it, someone probably does it in the bedroom. Heck, there are even those who get off by popping balloons (they're called looners). Everyone has at least one or two kinky desires, some more outrageous than others.

We encourage you to move forward with sensitivity and awareness. When evaluating a fantasy, kink, or fetish, be sure to ask yourself: Is it safe, sane, and consensual? If the answer to all three is yes, then it's up to you to decide whether to go with it! Keep in mind that once something is said, it can never be unsaid—as Dr. Glenda reminds us, the proverbial cat is out of the bag. So even if you talk about things that the two of you will never actually act on, we stress the importance of treating one another with respect and tenderness. A negative reaction can steer your sex life off course, and it can take a whole lot of extra work to get back to where you want to be.

Chapter **12**

GO FORTH AND F*CK

NOW THAT YOU ARE ARMED with important knowledge about those sexy creatures we call men, we hope you will use it. Remember, the most important elements of being a good lover and mastering your man are communication, creativity, self-respect, respect for your partner, true regard for your pleasure and his, and a sense of fun and adventure! In the spirit of play—sex play, that is—this chapter is filled with exercises that will help you put your new knowledge to work. We wish you a lifetime of great sex and outstanding orgasms, for the both of you.

END NOTES

[1] "Want to know if size really matters?" *Universities Australia*. Victoria University. 18 Aug. 2008. Web. 19 Nov. 2009.
www.universitiesaustralia.edu.au/database/news.asp?a=archive.

[2] Shah, J., and N. Christopher. "Can shoe size predict penile length?" *BJU International*. 90.6 (2002): 586–87. Print.

[3] Lyons, Andrew P., and Harriet D. Lyons. *Irregular Connections A History of Anthropology and Sexuality (Critical Studies in the History of Anthropology)*. New York: University of Nebraska, 2004. Print. p. 29.

[4] "The Kinsey Institute—Reference—Bibliographies—Penis Size [Related Resources]." *The Kinsey Institute for Research in Sex, Gender, and Reproduction*. Apr. 2009. Web. 20 Nov. 2009. www.kinseyinstitute.org/resources/bib-penis.html.

[5] "Detailed Tables—B02001. RACE—Universe: TOTAL POPULATION." *American FactFinder*. U.S. Census Bureau. Web. 29 Nov. 2009. http://factfinder.census.gov.

[6] Mayo Foundation for Medical Education and Research (MFMER), 1998–2009.

[7] *History of Circumcision*. Robert Darby, B.A., B.Litt., Ph.D. Web. 29 Nov. 2009.
www.historyofcircumcision.net/index.php?option=com_content&task=view&id=31&Itemid=54.

[8] Mika, ICCE, CD, Sheryl. *Better Birth Partners*. Web. 29 Nov. 2009. www.betterbirthpartners.com/NoCirc.html.

[9] Sorrells, Morris L., James L. Snyder, Mark D. Reiss, Christopher Eden, Marilyn F. Milos, Norma Wilcox, and Robert S. Van Howe. "Fine-touch pressure thresholds in the adult penis." *BJU International*. 99.4 (2007): 864–69. Print.

[10] Payne, Kimberley, Lea Thaler, Tuuli Kukkonen, Serge Carrier, and Yitzchak Binik. "Sensation and Sexual Arousal in Circumcised and Uncircumcised Men." *Journal of Sexual Medicine*. 4.3 (2007): 667–74. Print.

[11] "Testicles—Testicle Sperm Production." *Human Anatomy Online | Human Anatomy Study | Interactive Human Anatomy*. Web. 26 Nov. 2009. www.innerbody.com/image_repo02/repo10.html.

[12] Strong, Bryan, William Yarber, Barbara Sayad, and Christine DeVault. *Human Sexuality Diversity in Contemporary America*. 6th ed. New York: McGraw-Hill Humanities/Social Sciences/Languages, 2006. Print. p. 110.

[13] Strong, Bryan. p. 114.

[14] Kerner, Ian. *Passionista: The Empowered Woman's Guide to Pleasuring a Man*. New York: Collins, 2008. Print. p. 21.

[15] Kerner, Ian. p. 21.

[16] Strong, Bryan p. 124.

[17] Sutton, M.D. "The Mavens' Word of the Day." Random House: Bringing you the best in nonfiction, and children's books. Random House. 17 Aug. 2000. Web. 09 Feb. 2009. www.randomhouse.com/wotd/index.pperl?date=20000817.

[18] Hitchens, Christopher. "As American as Apple Pie." *Vanity Fair. VanityFair.com*, July 2006. Web. 09 Feb. 2009. www.vanityfair.com/culture/features/2006/07/hitchens200607?currentPage=1.

[19] *Online Etymology Dictionary*. Douglas Harper, Nov. 2001. Web. 11 Jan. 2010. www.etymonline.com/index.php.

[20] "Deep throat Made Easy." Welcome to Ra-Hoor-Khuit Network. Ra-Hoor-Khuit Network. 26 Feb. 1997. Web. 09 Feb. 2009. www.rahoorkhuit.net/library/yoga/tantra/techniques/deep_throat_made_easy.html.

[21] Johnson, Martin. *Essential Reproduction*. New York: Wiley, 2007. Print.

[22] "Understanding STDs—the Basics." *WebMD*, WebMD, LLC. 1 Aug. 2005. Web. 09 Feb. 2009. www.webmd.com/sex-relationships/understanding-stds-basics.

[23] Kerner, Ian. p. 156.